Praise for *The Yoga Way*

D0454429

"We cherish the light that shines through our
often succumb to parenting from a place of stress, anxiety, and feeling
deficiency. In this wise and important book, Shakta Khalsa offers teachings
and yoga practices that help us in becoming a true mirror for our children's goodness and allow them to fully inhabit their aliveness and spirit."
—Tara Brach, PhD, leading Western teacher of Buddhist (mindfulness)
meditation, emotional healing, and spiritual awakening, and author of
Radical Acceptance and *True Refuge*

"What would the world be like if children were introduced to the spiritual aspects of yoga at a young age? This wonderful book builds a bridge
between adults and children that reflects the unity that is the true meaning of yoga. If you love yoga, or know a child who could benefit, this
book can be your guide."
—Anodea Judith, PhD, author of
Wheels of Life and *Anodea Judith's Chakra Yoga*

"Shakta's *The Yoga Way to Radiance* is an inspiring collection of stories
and wisdom from her practice as counselor, yoga teacher trainer for children, and parent. You could open this book to any page and find a solution, a reminder, a breathing practice that could help you come back to
yourself and be present for a child. Shakta reminds us that parenting is
about evolving *with* our children, which is savvy advice from one whose
life's work is dedicated to a mission of conscious parenting."
—Wah!, author of *Healing: A Vibrational Exchange*
and *Dedicating Your Life to Spirit*

"An epic book whose time has come. It will connect children and parents
like only yoga can. I highly recommend it for parents, teachers, therapists, and all who love children."
—Larry Payne PhD, co-author of international
bestseller *Yoga for Dummies*

"Congratulations, Shakta, for your wonderful mission! Children are the future of tomorrow and it's about time that we pay attention to their needs. Through this book, Shakta is doing exactly that, to help in this worthy cause. It is her amazing effort that will change our future. Through her wonderful and comprehensive work she imparts her lifetime of wisdom and experience to help to cultivate a happier and healthier future generation."

—Dr. Madan Bali, PhD, author of *Taming the Mind*;
founder and director of Yoga Bliss Research and Training Institute

"Scientific evidence shows that yoga improves us in a number of ways: physically on the body and breath, emotionally by enhancing self-regulation of emotion and stress, cognitively by increasing mind-body awareness/mindfulness, and spiritually through unitive/contemplative experiences that improve life meaning and purpose. It is a challenge to live a yoga lifestyle incorporating these changes, and even more of a challenge to incorporate yogic practices and principles into the adult-child relationship. This book clearly elucidates the yogic psychological/philosophical concepts and practical strategies to achieve this, thereby providing children with the life skills to excel as human beings."

—Sat Bir Singh Khalsa, PhD, assistant professor of medicine at Harvard Medical School; chief editor of the *International Journal of Yoga Therapy* and the textbook *The Principles and Practice of Yoga in Health Care*

THE YOGA
WAY TO
Radiance

About the Author

Shakta Khalsa is one of the world's leading experts on children and yoga, having worked with both since the mid-1970s. She is a parent, Montessori educator, and founder of Radiant Child Yoga, one of the most well-known training programs for children's yoga and mindfulness. She is a trained yoga professional at the highest level (ERYT-500) and was named one of the top five Kundalini Yoga teachers in the world by *Yoga Journal*. Shakta studied under the direct guidance of Yogi Bhajan, Master of Kundalini Yoga, and she's also the author of five yoga books, including *Fly Like a Butterfly: Yoga for Children* and *Kundalini Yoga*. Shakta lives in Northern Virginia with her husband and their animal companions. Visit her online at www.childrensyoga.com and www.shaktawrites.com.

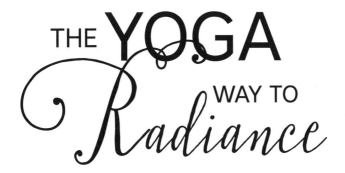

THE YOGA WAY TO Radiance

HOW TO FOLLOW YOUR INNER GUIDANCE AND NURTURE CHILDREN TO DO THE SAME

SHAKTA KHALSA

Llewellyn Publications
Woodbury, Minnesota

FIRST EDITION
First Printing, 2016

Cover art: iStockphoto.com/72260099/©altanaka
    iStockphoto.com/68624281/©homodans
Cover design: Ellen Lawson
Interior art: Mary Ann Zapalac
"Peace in Our Hearts, Peace in Our World: A Practice" by Shakta Khalsa in *Llewellyn's Complete Book of Mindful Living* © 2016 Llewellyn Worldwide, Ltd. 2143 Wooddale Drive, Woodbury, MN 55125. All rights reserved, used by permission.

Llewellyn Publications is a registered trademark of Llewellyn Worldwide Ltd.

Library of Congress Cataloging-in-Publication Data
Names: Khalsa, Shakta Kaur.
Title: The yoga way to radiance : how to follow your inner guidance and
    nurture children to do the same / by Shakta Khalsa.
Description: First Edition. | Woodbury : Llewellyn Worldwide, Ltd, 2016. |
    Includes bibliographical references.
Identifiers: LCCN 2016018665 (print) | LCCN 2016025634 (ebook) | ISBN
    9780738747767 | ISBN 9780738749679 ()
Subjects: LCSH: Yoga. | Parenting—Religious aspects—Yoga. | Child
    rearing—Religious aspects—Yoga.
Classification: LCC BL1238.54 .K43 2016 (print) | LCC BL1238.54 (ebook) | DDC
    204/.36—dc23
LC record available at https://lccn.loc.gov/2016018665

Llewellyn Worldwide Ltd. does not participate in, endorse, or have any authority or responsibility concerning private business transactions between our authors and the public.

All mail addressed to the author is forwarded but the publisher cannot, unless specifically instructed by the author, give out an address or phone number.

Any Internet references contained in this work are current at publication time, but the publisher cannot guarantee that a specific location will continue to be maintained. Please refer to the publisher's website for links to authors' websites and other sources.

Llewellyn Publications
A Division of Llewellyn Worldwide Ltd.
2143 Wooddale Drive
Woodbury, MN 55125-2989
www.llewellyn.com

Printed in the United States of America

Other Works by Shakta Khalsa

Yoga in Motion DVD
(2008)

Cozy CD
(2006)

Happy CD
(2006)

Yoga For Women
(DK Publishing, 2001)

K.I.S.S. Guide to Yoga
(DK Publishing, 2001)

Kundalini Yoga
(DK Publishing, 2001)

The Five Fingered Family
(Brookfield Reader, 2000)

Fly Like a Butterfly: Yoga for Children
(Sterling, 1999)

Yoga Warrior Cards

Acknowledgments

My deep gratitude to my long-time soul partner and husband, Kartar, who consistently holds a space of deep love and steady support for me and my work. I am so very thankful for our remarkable son, Ram Das, whose good nature has allowed me to use real-life examples from our relationship in this book, as well as in the Radiant Child Yoga program for these past decades.

I'd also like to acknowledge and thank Yogi Bhajan, who first opened my eyes to the soul of children, and to Maria Montessori, whose spirit continues to mentor me in my work. My deep thanks goes out to everyone at Llewellyn Publications, especially Angela Wix, Andrea Neff, and Vanessa Wright. Special thanks to Jill McKellan for creative writing support. And finally, to all friends and students whose stories appear in the book, to the dedicated Radiant Child Yoga facilitators, and to all who love children, I offer deep thanks and love.

Contents

Figures . . . xv

Foreword . . . xvii

Introduction: The Yoga Way to Radiance . . . 1

Personal Self, Greater Self   2

Healthy Attachment   3

An Invitation to Your Self   4

My Journey Toward My True Self   5

True Yoga from the Inside Out   9

Dedicated to All Who Love Children   10

Chapter 1: Welcome to Your Toolbox . . . 11

Real-Life Stories   12

How to Use This Book   14

Core Themes in Each Chapter   15

About Kundalini Yoga   17

Give Yoga a Chance   18

Chapter Highlights   19

Chapter 2: The Highest Path of Yoga . . . 21

Closing the Gap: Entering a Child's Mind   23

Finding the Gifts in the Challenges   25

The Energy Between Us   26

Fathering from the Soul: Kartar's Perspective   29

Being at Zero: A Practice   32

Breath as Sensation: A Practice   33

Experiencing Pure Awareness: A Practice   34

For Children: The Feather Breath   35

Chapter Highlights   36

Chapter 3: Walking the Balance Beam . . . 39

Light Energy   39

Logic and Respect   41

Tending to Our Tendencies   42

Parenting Karma   44

The Three Minds   49

The Compassion of the Neutral Mind   51

Practice: Sa Ta Na Ma Meditation   53

Children's Practice: Downdog and Bear Walk   56

Chapter Highlights   60

Chapter 4: Into the High Heart . . . 63

Directing Your Energy   63

The Effortless Effort   66

Recognizing Moments of Power   66

Creating Heart Space   68

The "Wouldn't It Be Wonderful If" Game   72

Loyal Friends: Breath and Imagination   73

Waves of Appreciation: A Practice   75

Heart-Opening Relaxation: A Practice   76

Yoga in Motion: Children's Practice   77

Chapter Highlights   82

Chapter 5: No Place Like Home . . . 83

First, Make Friends with Yourself   85

Our Child-Self Is Love: A Practice   88

Embracing Natural Cycles of Change   89

Being Outranks Doing: A Practice   93

The Only Opinion That Matters Is Yours   94

Letting Go of Parental Agenda   96

Getting Off the Momentum Machine   97

Staying Close to Home   99

Mindful Moments   101

Creating New Neural Pathways   102

Moving Out of the Old and Into the New: A Practice   103

Meditation: Stress Relief and Clearing Emotions from
the Past   108

Children's Practice: Butterfly-Cocoon   109

Chapter Highlights   111

Chapter 6: The Wonderful Side of Being Different . . . 113

Children with Special Intentions   114

Helpful Guidelines for Parents and Caregivers   121

Find the Fascination   124

Grounding Gifted Children   125

Understanding Our Needs   126

Diverse Souls within One Universe   128

Raising Your Energy Flow: A Practice   130

Bundle Roll Children's Practice   133

Log Roll: A Yoga Story   134

Chapter Highlights   136

Chapter 7: Giving Children Space to Grow . . . 137

Emotions in Flow   138

Staying Steady Through Emotional Times   140

Being a Non-Anxious Presence   143

Parenting from the Heart, Not the Hurts   145

Attention Without Apprehension   148

Letting Children Learn from Life   149

The Stories We Tell Ourselves   150

Natural Discipline   153

The Lighthearted Approach   156

Switchback Breath: A Practice   158

Journaling in Relation to Children: A Practice   160

I Am Happy Meditation: Children's Practice   161

Chapter Highlights   168

Chapter 8: Be the Lighthouse for Our Children, Our World . . . 169

Chakras and Children   170

Holding a Healing Space for a Child   172

Don't Bite the Bait!   176

Recognize You in the Other   176

Illuminating Our Dark Corners   177

Stepping Stones for Troubled Water   180

Raising the Lantern for the Next Generation   182

Radiating the Frequency of Peace   184

Peace in Our Hearts, Peace in Our World: A Practice   185

Chapter Highlights   188

Epilogue: In the Hands of the Universe . . . 189

Resources . . . 191

Figures

3a: Sa Ta Na Ma mudras   55

3b: Downdog   57

3c: Bear Walk   58

3d: Child's Pose   59

4a: Heart-Opening Relaxation   77

4b1 and 4b2: "I am brave!"   78

4c: "I am bold!"   79

4d: "My own spirit"   80

4e: "I can hold!"   81

5a: Cat Stretch   104

5b: Bridge Pose   105

5c: Knee Tuck   106

5d: Rock   107

5e: Meditation   108

5fa: Cocoon Pose   109

5fb: Butterfly Pose   110

6a: Sat Kriya   130

6b: Child's Pose   132

6c: Relaxation on back   132

6d: Bundle Roll   133

6e: Low Branch Tree   134

6f: High Branch Tree   135

7a: Switchback Breath   159

7b: "I am happy, I am good."   162

7c: "I am" (first)   163

7d: "I am" (second)   163

7e: "I am" (third)   164

7f: "Free!"   165

7g: "Happy, happy, happy to be"   166

7h: "Me!"   167

Disclaimer

The publisher and the author assume no liability for any injuries caused to the reader that may result from the reader's use of content contained in this publication and recommend common sense when contemplating the practices described in the work.

Foreword

We are beginning to understand the depth of experience our bodies give us regarding our world and those individuals we share this beautiful planet with. Those bodily experiences (which many scientists now call "consciousness" and even "cognition"), built from the beliefs and actions of our parents (even before birth), family, culture, and the world at large, determine our beliefs and reality. And the thoughts and feelings derived from that reality inform what we experience, and how we feel, nurture, and trust our own inner guidance. How we align with our own authentic selves, honoring our unique expression in this lifetime, will determine how our children mirror us and step into their own power as unique expressions, honoring, trusting, and following their own inner guidance, or not.

In this highly informative and heart-centered book, Shakta Khalsa views caring for children as the highest path of yoga. Shakta encourages each parent, each grandparent, and everyone working with children to first step into their own authentic selves in order to reflect that authenticity to the children they nurture. In every chapter, she provides stories, meditations, energy work, and yoga activities that assist us to remember and live from our inner place of truth, being our own light and the light for those around us.

We know from scientific research that when we follow our instincts, intuition, or what my friend Antony Trowbridge calls our "In Tutor," we will be over 90 percent correct in our thoughts and actions. Shakta, with great clarity and profound meditations, yoga, and inner work, guides us to feel, trust, and follow our own inner guidance again ... as we did as children. She sees children as our teachers when they are free to truly express their wonder, curiosity, and deep delight with their world. We know, from Rivlin and Gravel's work at Princeton University, that there are far more than the five senses we have been taught we function from. There are at least nineteen senses that we know of receptor sites for, and probably hundreds that we haven't understood yet. Our children are fully aware, using all their senses to understand the world around them. They mirror us in the process of learning to be human. And they sense all that we are thinking and feeling, way beyond our words. Our being authentic allows them to trust their senses of us, and in so doing, to learn empathy, compassion, and altruism.

What I truly love about this book is its ability to bring me home to myself—over and over. As I read it, each chapter and lesson touched my heart and reminded me again to come home to me in order to be fully present to all those around me—especially children, who are acutely aware of my energies and who challenge me to be authentic, real, and honest with them, sharing my whole being so they can fully share all that they are. So often, as parents, or when working with children, we feel we must control their actions so they are always safe, responsible, well mannered, and—in short—reflections of what we believe (from our take on reality) will make them easily fit in to the world. In so doing, we also put those restrictions on our own lives and lose the ability to be fully present and authentic in each moment. We stop the flow of our gifts to the world and also stop the spontaneity of our children to show us new horizons and, more importantly, their gifts.

Shakta Khalsa has provided us with a doorway that leads back home to ourselves, in order to step into our own power, trusting everyone else (including our children) to step into their own power. *The Yoga Way to Radiance* provides valuable tools to assist us in embracing our inner guidance, expressing our unique beings, learning each moment, living with wonder and joy, and mirroring that to our children and the world. May you gain a joyful sense of authenticity as you step through the doorway of this book.

Carla Hannaford, PhD, author of *Awakening the Child Heart: Handbook for Global Parenting* and *Playing in the Unified Field: Raising and Becoming Conscious, Creative Human Beings*

INTRODUCTION

The Yoga Way to Radiance

During the late 1980s and after a decade of wanting to have a child, my husband, Kartar, and I sought guidance from our spiritual teacher, Yogi Bhajan, a fiercely passionate and compassionate yoga master from India whose vision of an enlightened humanity had led him west to share his knowledge.

In dealing with strong emotions that were catalyzed by our deep longing, we had been counseled over the years to do particular meditations or to relax and let it come to us. One personal letter that I received from Yogi Bhajan simply said, "Love God." I took that to mean relax and accept, and in the accepting, something good could happen. But time moved on and there was still no child. For me, this translated into anxiety at best and deep pain at worst.

The day came for our meeting with Yogi Bhajan. I remember crowds of people around us on every side as we waited for our turn to have an audience with him. Kartar and I sat at the foot of the beautifully decorated platform and equally majestic presence of the teacher. With as much presence as we could muster, we asked for his help. He looked directly into my eyes with a piercing gaze that entered into my soul. It seemed that gaze held for at least a minute. He spoke one sentence only: "Why do you want to have a child?"

I don't remember if I even answered him. I was acutely aware that it wasn't a question meant to be answered or have a dialogue about. He was giving me a koan—a puzzle that has no real answer because it is meant to enlighten. It shook me on the spot. I felt in his gaze and in his words a timeless idea that was just out of reach—a key to my hope and misery.

Personal Self, Greater Self

I went home with that moment echoing in my insides. I was shaken in a way that could only be handled through deep meditation and contemplative inquiry through journaling. As his question resounded in my mind and heart, I felt the emptiness of each of my answers—even though to the normal human world, my answers seemed sensible, logical, and natural: *I want to have a child to love. I want to have the happiness of being a mother. I want the deep satisfaction of having a child who came from my husband's and my deep connection to each other and to the spiritual path. I want to bring in a child who will help bring this world into an age of peace and harmony.*

But now my teacher's gaze and his powerful words awakened the soul within me. Somehow his words had touched the depth of my inner being, which then seemed to stand before me in response to my litany of beliefs. There was an instant knowing of the place—the edge—where each of the "truths" that I believed showed themselves to be untrue. Each reason that I presented was undone by an immediate sense of knowing from the soul level...

Me (as personal self): *I want a child to love. I want the happiness of being a mother.*

Me (as greater Self): *You know your happiness doesn't depend on anything. And if you think it depends on being a mother, you'll end up relying on the child for your fulfillment—not a good reason to bring in a child.*

And so it went. The overall feeling of the internal conversation I was having became something like this: *We both know the limitations of this way of thinking. It is a nice story, but it is still a story. And can you understand how that story is the source of misery?*

Healthy Attachment

All the wise sages throughout time have talked about nonattachment being the key to happiness. I don't believe they are trying to say that you shouldn't adore, love, and nurture your children. But I do believe they are saying that if you base your emotional satisfaction and your connection to spirit on your relationship with anyone—including your children—you will most likely experience pain when they disappoint you, because they are not born to serve anyone but their own spirit, as are you. When we try to derive our wellbeing and satisfaction from our children, or anyone else, it ends up being an unhealthy attachment, since no person other than ourselves can be our source of happiness and fulfillment. I believe Yogi Bhajan's potent question was helping me to come to that conclusion through my own power of insight.

Many years after this period of time, I came across Byron Katie's book *Loving What Is*. One of the four questions in her work echoed exactly the voice of my greater, authentic Self in saying, "Who would I be without that thought?" Without the thought that I should have a child, that I should be a mother, that it would ruin my idea of how my life should be if I weren't one—without those thoughts, I felt the first stirrings of freedom from inner pressure to have something I didn't have. For the first time in a long time, a sense of peacefulness began to settle around me. It was as if the corner of a large lead blanket had been lifted from my mind and heart. And so it was, temporarily. Then the anxiety would return, but less often and less powerfully.

Many months went by and the one simple unanswerable question dominated my world. Yet through deep meditation and authentic inquiry, what at first seemed like a ghost that haunted me day and night became increasingly more corporeal until the "ghost," my greater Self, became myself. Gradually and without fanfare, I felt a surrendering into the understanding that "there is no really good reason; it will be or it will not be." There was relief—punctuated by panic at times—but still, relief from allowing things to be steered into existence, or not, by the unknown hand of the universe.

More years passed, and more changes and internal growth helped to prepare me, at age forty-one and after fourteen years of marriage, to mother a very special son. The experience of deep inquiry into what it meant to be a parent was the first foot forward on the path of parenting, a path that never ends but continues to shift and evolve. We find that we are born together, parent and child, and we are always in the process of becoming.

An Invitation to Your Self

Through the pages of this book, I invite you to make friends with yourself and your child and step into a radiant flow of life. Here we'll create space to explore a new vision of our relationship with these bright souls that we call children. The words, images, and personal stories in this book are designed to help you step out of struggle, shrug off the "I shoulds," and breathe deeply again. Through the intimacy of soul-talk, I will speak to the you who knows; the radiant, authentic you; the You with a capital *Y*. Once you connect with You, it will be easier for your children to match that space of connection. Because, you see, they have an advantage—they haven't yet unlearned what they came here knowing: that they are powerful, radiant beings made of the same stuff as the Source they came from.

For now, get into the spirit by feeling the happy anticipation of what is to come: a tenderhearted spaciousness filled with rich, deep, joyful, ever-evolving life for you and your children.

In yoga, there is a greeting, *namaste*, which translates as "the light in me recognizes and honors the light in you." This is the place where we start our journey together. The underlying theme of every chapter in this book is centered on the idea of honoring, because no matter what idea or skill we are focusing on, we will always be honoring our authentic Selves and the authentic beings we call children.

My Journey Toward My True Self

Like many people, I grew up without a real sense of knowing what honoring felt like, or even what it really was. This was nobody's fault—my family did the best they could based on what they knew about life. They just didn't have helpful tools like yoga or understand that it was possible to live a happier, more authentic life, so they couldn't teach me how to do what they didn't know. It led to some challenges, something we all can relate to, but what I took away from my experiences was this: if I can turn my life around to be able to live more as my true, happy Self and honor that "self" in others, then I know that you can do it as well.

The stories of our lives are often long and complicated, so I want to share with you the short version of my journey toward my true self.

Because I've been immersed in the world of children and yoga for forty years, it may appear to you that my life has always been about children. This is not true. For the first twenty-five years of my life, it was about me—specifically, who I was in relation to others and who I was on the inside, when no one else was around. There was a distinct difference between the two, and I spent many years trying to reconcile them. The inside "me" is what I now think of as my authentic Self. Like a budding flower, my authentic Self gradually blossomed over those first decades of my life, nurtured through the water and sun of yoga, meditation, and inner awareness.

From the place where I now stand, I can see things more clearly. The strongest childhood memories I have are those in which I was consciously aware that through a challenging experience, I had the opportunity to understand the workings of the energy flow that we call "life." I did not think of it in those terms then, but I sensed a deeper meaning, knowing that what I was thinking and feeling dictated how I acted. In turn, this had a direct impact on the outcome. Here's a simple example. When I was a young teen, I enjoyed floating face down in my family's small above-ground backyard pool. I found it relaxing; it felt like my body didn't exist. One of my favorite things to do was to see how long

I could hold my breath as I floated, and I loved to count the seconds in my mind. I recall a particular time when I was aware of a pressurized feeling that indicated I needed to take a breath. I heard the thought, *I can't hold it any longer.* And then there was another part of me, one who had a bigger perspective, saying, *But you held it through that thought! And if you held it through that thought, then you can hold it through another.* With a feeling of amazement for my own inner wisdom, I emerged from the water for a breath only when I absolutely knew it was time.

In this story, I was clearly connected to my authenticity and received the confirmation that "things work out for me." Then there were the countless other times, those moments when I was in the mode of learning by trial and error. Today, just like yesterday, I am so grateful that I have been able to recognize that in every challenge there is a gift—and the bigger the challenge, the bigger the gift.

I was lucky enough to be a young adult in the early 1970s. With the "peace and love" attitude of my generation coupled with my abiding focus on how life works from the inside, I felt I had ended up where I was meant to be. During my college years, I was drawn to Eastern spiritual philosophy and practice, and as a result, four well-spent years passed with me sitting daily on my yoga blanket, practicing postures and meditations. This practice awakened my senses and helped guide me to understand what was true and right for me, and how to honor that feeling in myself and others. As you can imagine, this was so liberating! Everything just made a bit more sense to my logical mind, as well as in the way I felt internally.

In 1976 I was introduced to Kundalini yoga, which is often called the "quick-results yoga" because many people experience an immediate and ongoing rise in their ability to connect with their authentic Self. I remember my first class, and the way I felt my body becoming an instrument for moving internal energy toward enlightenment. I had the distinct feeling that my four years of solitary yoga practice had allowed me to graduate into the transformative experience of Kundalini Yoga as taught by Yogi Bhajan, who brought this yoga tradition from India to North America in 1968.

In the early days of yoga in the Western culture, it was often a *path* you took, not a *class* you took. The yogic lifestyle was a way of living, complete with a healthy plant-based diet, early morning practice, mindful communication between yourself and others, and an opportunity to live your yoga in every passing moment. During this time, spiritual communities called *ashrams* sprouted up across the nation and internationally as a way to support the yogic lifestyle. This was where I met my soon-to-be husband, Kartar, in the yoga ashram where we recognized that we were, and are, kindred souls and married in 1977.

After the adult morning practice in our community, everyone took turns leading the children's version of morning yoga. To my surprise and delight, I found that I had a real knack for creating playful yoga stories and sharing yogic understandings in ways that children could relate to. One special experience led to another, and soon I was sharing my newfound love for children and yoga in the Montessori school that the children attended. My love for these children and how I could help them start their beautiful lives more authentically kept growing. Soon I knew that my calling was to become a certified Montessori teacher.

In 1982 I started my own school, weaving yoga, meditation, guided relaxation, and conscious communication skills into the children's daily routine. I was constantly amazed at these small, brilliant beings that we call children. I would teach them something and feel like I was the one learning. Today, I can look back at that ten-year time period and recognize a subtle sense of taking an unspoken sacred vow to be a champion for children by becoming one who helps them maintain their connection to their authentic selves.

Besides running the school during the 1980s, Kartar and I had two children come to live with us, each for three years. It seemed that within the nationwide Kundalini yoga communities, Kartar and I had gotten a reputation as being a good resource for parents whose children were extremely challenging. We foster-parented a three-year-old girl who had screaming fits for hours at a time. Her mother moved to our community to learn from us, and gradually reclaimed the parenting role. Our next child was a four-year-old boy who was hyperactive (the label ADD/ADHD was not commonplace in those days). He had anger issues and was in great need of a father figure to look up to, which he found in Kartar. These two parenting experiences heightened my awareness of how the child's issues and the adult's issues were completely intertwined, whether the adult was the natural parent or not. I was grateful to know this and understand its importance. The real importance is in the realization that the intricate interplay that takes place between a child and an adult happens not just with parents, but also with relatives, caregivers, teachers, and therapists.

Having parenting experience was comforting, because in 1991 Kartar and I were overjoyed to become parents to a child, a son named Ram Das. While he was young, I began specializing in teaching children's yoga and very quickly had several schools and daycare centers that I traveled to each week, teaching upwards of five hundred children between the ages of three and ten. Parents and teachers were very responsive to what they saw from the children after these classes, and as a result, many people asked me to write a children's yoga book so they could continue to do yoga at home. This was the inspiration behind my first book, *Fly Like a Butterfly: Yoga for Children,* which was quickly followed by four more books, another one for children and three adult yoga books.

To put it in Montessori terms, I was in a "sensitive period" for writing for about five years, wanting to get all these incredible insights and yoga tools that I had become aware of down on paper. As the authoring period faded, I felt an unmistakable calling from my heart. Someone once said that the child is the root of the heart. Well, I could feel the root of my heart telling me to return to the work with children and those who care for them. As a result, in 1999 I founded a children's yoga training program, one of the first in the world, called Radiant Child Yoga. With a humble beginning of teaching a few parents and teachers with a simple manual and yoga book, the training has expanded considerably over the years to include tens of thousands of professionals as well as parents. During these sessions, participants receive a plethora of materials, including DVDs, CDs, and books to help them start out strong on their journey. Honestly, it's an honor to help adults find ways to help little beings grow up into people who are connected with their authentic selves. What a blessing for the future of our world! I've also learned so much from the various creative ways my students are working with children. You will hear from some of them throughout the pages of this book. Through this amazing effort, a joint venture of instructor and participant, Radiant Child Yoga became a Yoga Alliance accredited training school in 2009, at the 95- and 200-hour levels.

True Yoga from the Inside Out

I have come to realize that most people have not had early life training in how to be aware of themselves as energy beings with their own bona fide inner guidance. And as I said earlier, neither did I—not until I began deeply exploring the idea that how we feel and what we think inform what we experience. This is when I began having very clear experiences and manifestations of where our power resides, and that is in our ability to truly know ourselves. Many people find that yoga, including meditation and mindfulness, is one of the best ways to experience themselves as the powerful authentic beings that they are, so we'll be using these holistic tools throughout the book. I hope you will think of yoga as more than just a system to help you relax and release anxiety or tone your body, but also as a way of experiencing the oneness of everything—of ourselves as body, mind, and spirit, and of our relationship with others, including our children.

The deeper purpose of this book can be distilled into a few words: to learn how to feel, trust, and follow your own inner guidance and nurture children to do the same. This innate inner knowing is something we are all born with. Children are more easily able to live in their authentic selves since they haven't yet "unlearned" their natural connection to their inner guidance, making them wonderful reminders that they are teachers to us just as much as we are teachers to them.

Dedicated to All Who Love Children

This may seem like a parenting book, but it is not solely for parents. The intention is to honor all the relationships we have with children, so the ideas and experiences in *The Yoga Way to Radiance* are also relevant for teachers, therapists, and professionals who work with children. More than half of the tens of thousands of people I've worked with in my training program have been educators, therapists, and caregivers. In using these yoga tools and insights, they have experienced remarkable positive changes in the children they work with and in their interactions with them.

Anytime you align with your authentic Self and honor your unique expression, you will naturally know how to be present in situations that arise with children. This connection is your foundation. It is the touchstone for your relationship with children. I'll give you stories, insights, tips, and tools along the way to help you recognize moments of opportunity to positively impact children. Also, there are many wonderfully effective books available that provide words and skills to deal with behavior. You will find a list of them in the resources section of this book, should you care to draw from them.

And so, friends, as we embark on this exciting journey, living from our inner place of truth for our own benefit as well as the benefit of our children, I bow to you again, with *namaste* and a reminder that the journey, once started, never ends. But that is good news; there is always more to learn about being authentic, being the light, and honoring ourselves and everyone else. On our journey, the child shines the light to show us the way home.

CHAPTER 1

Welcome to Your Toolbox

In understanding the structure of our work together, it may be helpful to think of each chapter in this book as an individual facet of a bright diamond. Each facet shines its own light, one that is focused on a particular aspect of creating a happy life within ourselves and with our children. While these facets are equally important to the glow of the diamond, you may find that some of them resonate with you more than others, and that is okay. Oftentimes when things resonate within us, it is our guidance telling us *yes!* I also feel an inner warmth from whatever resonates with me, reminding me of how our happiness radiates outward from within us.

Within each chapter, you will embark on an experiential journey into the way you currently view your relationship with your children. You may also gain insight into your own childhood, both the delights and the challenges, and begin to transform the parts of your relationship with children that you would like to be happier, to be more true to who you feel you both are. This is the journey we will be taking together, and the benefits are many, including the following:

- Learning ancient wisdom that is congruent with leading-edge thought to guide you and your child to be the radiant, authentic beings that you truly are

- Making friends with yourself by honoring wherever you are on your journey, then seeing how the act of honoring is also fostered in your child

- Practicing processes to help you either reconnect with or remain connected to your authentic Self while meeting challenges with children

- Practicing fun and effective yoga and meditation exercises that will help guide you and your child to a place of balance, as well as assist you in integrating the themes of each chapter into practical and applicable actions

- Accessing an inner place of trust in your child's natural self-correcting abilities and inner guidance by acknowledging and understanding that you can also trust these same abilities in yourself

Real-Life Stories

You are invited into the world of real people—friends, students, and trainers for my program—who have been using the ideas in this book with results that border on miraculous. With gratitude to all of the courageous souls who are practicing an extraordinary life within themselves and with children, here is our first story to inspire you onward!

Samir and Jyoti grew up in an Indian culture where yoga and meditation were part of daily life. Still, living as Westerners with busy multitasking lives had caused them to put their yoga roots aside. Some years ago, however, both Jyoti and Samir began working with Law of Attraction energy-based work, which included nightly meditation. Along with their young teen son, Akshay, they began a consistent routine, knowing that repetition is important for keeping old patterns at bay. If Samir and Jyoti got busy and didn't initiate the nightly gathering, Akshay would keep the family on track. Samir recounted with a beaming face, "We want our children to have tools to stay positive, and not just tell them to stay positive. When we are not doing it, they think, 'Well, you are not doing it, so why should I do it?' At one point I was taking the lead in keeping our nightly meditation going, and Akshay was the lieutenant. He would say, 'You got to keep doing it, Papa.' He was showing his love for me through this. He was showing me how much he loves me and wants me to feel good. Now I am choking up!"

Jyoti chimed in: "It has been such a wonderful experience to bring us all closer. Now, it may be the same situation, but we look at it differently. Instead of being reactionary, we just see what opportunities are available to us." Jyoti then gave an example of how the nightly meditation and inner energy work had helped them to discover natural discipline and trust in their son's ability to rise to whatever challenge presented itself.

She went on: "We had some real homework struggles in the pre-teen years, before we started this daily commitment to meditation. I used to get so stressed-out over making sure he was studying and doing homework. I would hover over him and fuss about it. I made a chart—a homework timetable—but it didn't help. There was also a struggle about getting to school on time, with me pushing him to get ready. After some time of working internally with these issues, a new insight dawned on me: I really understood that I don't have control over other people and situations and only have control over my own thoughts, actions, and emotions. With that insight, I felt myself relax more. Instead of working on changing him, I started to observe myself so I could be a better parent."

Jyoti's voice became lighter and clearer as she recounted what happened next. "At one point, I sat down with Akshay and apologized to him. I told him that I was not going to insist on using the timetable, which didn't work anyway because it was made by me. I sincerely wanted to handle it differently. I saw the possibility of using our meditative minds together, and this was the attitude that opened it up for both of us. He was looking at me in amazement. I told him that at 7:50 a.m. I would be ready to take him to school. At first, he was consistently late, but I just trusted that natural consequences would be the teacher for him. I would just take him whenever he was ready rather than bugging him. After a week of being late, he announced that it didn't make him feel good to be the last one in the class. So I asked him what time he needed to get up to make it work. He figured it out and set his alarm, and that was the last time he was late. I didn't have to start my day screaming. It resolved because the solution came from him.

"I stopped interfering with his homework. After a while of just doing whatever he wanted, he was not getting his homework done. It was hard to watch this, but I left it alone, again, just trusting that it would work out. Akshay came to me one night and said, 'I need your help in lesson planning and management.' We sat down and made a timetable together. I was just following his lead. He knew that he needed down-time when he got home, so every day he had that on the schedule. His grades came back up, and he still manages his schedule all by himself."

Samir brought the story back around to the inner work: "Some of my best teachers talk about letting things go, because the more you struggle against something, the more powerful it gets. This attitude has become our family's baseline in everyday life. For example, once when I was upset with Akshay I said, 'I am your dad!' His immediate response was, 'But you don't own me.' Instead of being reactive, I thought, *Oh my gosh, he knows this! And after forty years I am just learning this. I really don't own him. He is a person in his own right, and my job is to guide him and to truly see that he has his own guidance.*"

How to Use This Book

With this family's story, it becomes apparent that it is possible to reclaim our own authenticity and nurture the same in our children. Toward that end, here are some tips on how to make the most of what you find in these pages:

- Read this book as if you were reading a good book of poetry or prose, slowly and thoughtfully. Let the ideas sink in, then test them out in real life.

• As you go through the book, allow yourself to be okay with ideas you don't understand or agree with. If you can begin to meet confused or conflicting feelings with a relaxed and "trusting the universe" attitude, you are more likely to gain insight and solutions that become beacons of light for your unique expression of inner guidance.

• At the end of each chapter, there are experiential practices to ground the themes contained in that chapter. Where appropriate, these adult practices have been adapted for children. There is also a practice specifically oriented toward children ages three through ten at the end of each chapter. I encourage you to enjoy your relationship with your child in new ways through playful and meaningful yoga. Through this, I believe you will experience you and your child opening up and connecting in ways that would not normally happen in the flow of regular everyday life. If you find that your child is resisting your invitation to do yoga, don't be attached to an outcome. Just do it yourself, and if your child sees you enjoying it, he or she may decide to join you.

• Take advantage of the chapter summaries, which reiterate the messages and concepts covered in the chapter, helping you to remember key ideas and embrace them as your journey begins.

Core Themes in Each Chapter

Each chapter is threaded with underlying insights to ponder. As you read each chapter, I suggest you pause at sections where you see this mark: ***. Put down the book and take a breath, as this will allow deeper insights to settle within your consciousness. Be in a space where you are open to whatever life brings to you. The following core themes repeat throughout the book:

• Mindfully checking in with yourself in the moment

• Noticing "what is" without pushing away thoughts or feelings, nor following them wherever they may lead

- Developing and trusting your intuition as you choose inner processes and outer practices
- Making note of new insights mentally, verbally, or through journaling

Inner Processes: Each chapter will focus on a variety of helpful processes, such as using positive self-talk, being fully present and fully neutral, seeing the gifts in challenges, learning to trust inner guidance, becoming aware of how thoughts and feelings create reality, and, most importantly, learning to be an example of authenticity for the children in your life.

Outer Practices: Many people who practice yoga do so to maintain their health and wellbeing, improve physical fitness, relieve stress, and enhance their quality of life. In addition, they may be addressing specific health conditions, such as back pain, neck pain, arthritis, or anxiety. Yoga has also proven to be an essential practice for many adults who are looking for ways to deepen their mind-body connection.

It's quite natural that the benefits of yoga practice would carry over to children too, and the studies show it! According to two 2015 reports by researchers from the National Center for Health Statistics and the National Institutes of Health, yoga was the most used mind-body practice in 2012, with 9.5 percent of American adults (21 million) and 3.1 percent of children (1.7 million) using yoga that year.[1] I find it exciting to see how fast children's yoga is growing: 429,000 more children used yoga in 2012 than in 2007.

These studies show what hundreds of my friends and students have confirmed, as well as what I have experienced. Individuals who choose and embrace a regular practice of yoga and meditation can facilitate their own ability to become happier, healthier, and more aligned with their true Self.

---

1. National Center for Complementary and Integrative Health, "Use of Complementary Health Approaches in the US: Most Used Mind and Body Practices," February 10, 2015, https://nccih.nih.gov/research/statistics/NHIS/2012/mind-body/yoga.

About Kundalini Yoga

With a regular practice of yoga and meditation, you may find yourself connecting with others in ways that are soul-satisfying. Yoga and meditation tools will help your internal transformation become self-evident and stabilized.

Yoga

Based in Kundalini Yoga as taught by Yogi Bhajan, this powerful and quite doable system of yoga includes postures (asanas) and exercises (kriyas) coupled with rhythmic breathing patterns. Kundalini Yoga includes using sound (mantra), breathwork (pranayama), and meditative internal awareness. Here are some good things to know before you begin your practice:

- Before starting Kundalini Yoga and meditation, sit on the floor with your legs crossed at the ankles. This is called Easy Pose. You can use a pillow or blanket, if necessary, to help straighten the lower spine. Alternatively, you may sit on a straight-backed chair. Lift your breastbone and straighten your neck so your chin is level with the floor and slightly tucked. This allows the spinal fluid and the internal energy (prana) to flow through the spine and into the brain and body.

- Press the palms of the hands together at the center of the chest (heart center) and chant the "tune-in" mantra, *Ong Namo Guru Dev Namo*, three times—once for each deep breath. If you are in an environment where chanting is discouraged, tune in with the mantra out loud before entering the environment, then tune in to start the practice with three deep breaths. *Ong Namo* means "I honor the entire universe," and *Guru Dev Namo* means "I recognize the great guidance, the light that exists within me and all around me."

- You are welcome to end your Kundalini Yoga and meditation session with the traditional ending "The Long Time Sun." If you don't know the melody to this song, you may just say the words to yourself or out loud as a beautiful blessing for yourself and others: *May the long time sun shine upon you, all love surround you. And the pure light within you, guide your way on.*

- Children's yoga based in Kundalini Yoga is generally dynamic and playful. You may like to use creative storytelling to go along with the yoga postures and exercises. Many such stories can be found in my book *Fly Like a Butterfly: Yoga for Children.*

- Invite the child to do yoga with you, and make it fun while remembering the parts that keep it yoga: focus, breath, and inner connection. Taking a big breath at the end of each pose helps draw in the focus. Remember, children "play" at yoga. Let them practice yoga as they are able, no matter how imperfect it may seem from an adult point of view.

Meditation

Kundalini Yoga contains a wealth of valuable meditations, and in this book you'll find several that are relevant to the themes being explored. Instructions for mental focus, eye focus, and hand position (mudra) are given within the context of each individual meditation.

Journaling

Where appropriate, you will be invited to reflect on questions and then journal in order to deepen the experience of reflection.

Give Yoga a Chance

The tools in this book are not complicated; they are simple and they work for those who apply them. As you read through the chapters, consider giving a few minutes a day to whichever of these processes and practices speak to you. One great suggestion for delving more deeply into the transformative sections of the book is to choose one process, or a yoga and meditation practice, and work with it for one week, for twenty minutes to an hour each day, as you are able. Many people find that starting the day with a combination of yoga and meditation puts them on the path to an extraordinary day, week, year, and life!

Aside from the concepts in this book being sound tools for connecting with inner guidance and happiness, they are also natural and portable, and, most importantly, they work if you work with them! Countless people throughout the ages have used yoga, meditation, journaling, inner awareness, and mindfulness to create and maintain a connection with themselves, with children, and with their greater Selves. The amazing things that can happen when we share the gifts of awareness with children are beyond what we can fathom. From decades of working with adults and children with these tools, I've noticed that the biggest challenge for many is to open their mind and embrace the notion of giving these awareness tools a chance, both for their own sake and for the sake of the children they love. Most of us would do anything for a child. While we can't do everything for them, we can ensure that we are giving them sustainable gifts that, if they choose to use them, will serve them throughout their lives.

Chapter Highlights

- **Honoring:** In this book we will endeavor to honor all the ways of being that children and adults choose to express, and thereby find the gift in each expression.

- **Helpful tools:** By consistently doing yoga, meditation, and inner energy work, there is the opportunity for the mind, body, and spirit to harmonize, creating an extraordinary life of living in the natural wisdom of the authentic Self.

- **Joyful life:** When things feel complicated, let's go back to the basics and realize that our overarching purpose in this work is simply to make life easier and happier for ourselves and those in our care.

CHAPTER 2
The Highest Path of Yoga

Parenting has been called "the highest path of yoga," and for good reason. Where else do you have the challenge and the opportunity to be at your most mindful in each moment? Where else does your every communication have the potential to create conflict or to uplift?

Let's talk about energy. We often say that we wish we had as much energy as children have. In this context, we are referring to the lively, kinetic, sometimes frenetic energy that children can display. While we can envy this high level of energy and are often at a loss for what to do with it (more about that later in the chapter), the type of energy we're focusing on here is also referred to as *life force energy*. In yoga, it's called *prana*, and in Qi Gong, it's *qi*. It flows through us, around us, and between us, and from a molecular level perspective, we are energy beings. Our internal energy is affected by the way we feel, which is affected by the way we think and what we believe.

Children respond both consciously and unconsciously to everything happening in each moment of their day and are more attuned to the "feeling-energy" of each moment than we adults are. A positive illustration of this comes from my friend Amy. She lives by the ocean and spends a lot of time at the beach with her three young children. One day she had a remarkable experience with her two-and-a-half-year-old son,

Fisher. In her words: "I was sitting on the beach with Fisher in my lap, helping him eat his popsicle. He had just woken up from a nap when we got to the beach, so he was quiet and peaceful, happy to just sit with me as I was holding his popsicle so he could enjoy its yumminess. The girls were playing happily, creating a 'dance show' a little bit away from me. I felt so happy—happy kids, sun shining, waves crashing … everything felt just right. I began to internally acknowledge, *Thank you, thank you, thank you.* Not a moment later, Fisher hopped up out of my lap and began to dance around, yelling out loud, 'Thank you, thank you, thank you!' Amazing! Energy-love shared and expressed."

Yes, as anyone who has been around babies can testify, children come into life with a natural sense of being. As long as their basic needs are met, they are purely radiant and present. Their absorbent minds pick up feelings and ways of thinking from those around them. These ways of thinking become habits, and for better or worse, they influence the child from day one onward. Whether you are a parent or a caregiver, life with children can run the gamut from exhilaration, as in Amy's story, all the way to habitual discord and conflict.

When it comes to the topic of conflict, I am reminded of one of my students, a sixth grade teacher named Sarah. In her children's yoga training with me, she learned a breathing technique called the Feather Breath. She immediately felt that this could be the key with one of her students, a boy named Kevin who had sensory integration challenges and could become violent when he got frustrated because he didn't understand something. Sometimes Sarah had to move all the children to one corner of the room for safety because he would throw chairs when he was in a rage. She reported that she introduced the Feather Breath technique to Kevin when he was receptive and calm. She encouraged him to hold the feather by his face and blow on it hard to make it bend. Blowing on the feather allowed Kevin to oxygenate his blood, get his brain unstuck from patterns, and release strong emotions that were pent up inside. Sarah reports that this simple technique has been the key to bringing order and calm to the classroom, and that Kevin is now able to recognize when strong emotion is welling up and actually asks for the feather! This type of success, even if it's with only one child, is exciting because it demonstrates one of countless natural and intuitive ways to *help children help themselves.*

It is to Sarah's credit that she recognized Kevin's need and trusted his ability to self-regulate if given the right tools. Rather than reacting to a potentially dangerous situation, she had the presence of mind to try out a creative solution. This is not easy to do, as any parent or teacher can attest! Being around children can make us painfully aware of our gaps in awareness. Much of the time, we adults have taken on a more left-brain approach, which doesn't give us access to creative solutions. Often we have dulled our sensitivity to the flow of energy between us all and, sadly, to our own intuitive capacity. But the good news is that children and adults alike have the same essence, and we can find our way back to our essential nature again and again.

Closing the Gap: Entering a Child's Mind

As an adult, I know I have many gaps in awareness, times when I am just functioning from my habitual mind. When I want to be more present to myself or to a child, I have found it helpful to remember what it feels like to have a child's mind. When I recall how I thought or felt as a child, it seemed that I had understandings beyond those that were exhibited by the adults in my family. Even though these thoughts and feelings were not fully formed, I unconsciously sensed that I understood life differently. I had a private world that was filled with wonder and kindness. I felt as if the whole universe were smiling down on me and guiding me along, that everyone had the same connection to this wonderful energy that I did, because we are all made of the same stuff. Animals, trees, plants, and the loving feelings that emanated from my family toward me were touchstones for something that I knew deep within me: we are good, we are born in goodness, and we are shining lights of love … born in radiance.

***

Since young children have not yet developed the qualities of self-reflection and self-awareness, most of our early memories are vague and subtle. They are more felt than consciously understood. It is possible, however, to have an experience that is life-changing enough to "flash" an imprint in our awareness, even at a young age. I had an experience like this, and it was a poignant, defining moment in my life.

When I was four years old, I had an experience that has remained with me as a conscious moment in time. I can still recall the scenario and dialogue and, most importantly, the flash of understanding that occurred in my four-year-old brain. I was at a family gathering at my grandparents' house. The food was set out buffet-style on the table. I was looking at my uncle when my mother's voice pierced the moment, saying, "Do you want another chicken leg?" With a shock, I saw that my uncle was holding a piece of food in his right hand—a piece of food that before that moment was just "food" to me, but then it became an actual chicken's leg. I saw the shape of it, and in my mind, I matched it with an image of a chicken running around on her two legs. The image turned into a feeling of dreadful pain. I realized for the first time that meat is animals' bodies.

From day one, animals had always been my best friends during my childhood. My own beloved dog, Stubby, was born around the same time that I was and was my only companion until my sister was born five years later. Stubby and I shared looks that needed no words. If I needed to use words, she was always there to listen and make things better. Somehow the magical connection between animals and me extended to all types of animals, from bugs to birds to cats to frogs. They were more true and natural than the adults around me. I understood them, and they understood me. I didn't even think of them as "animals"; they were just friends—from the spider carefully collected in a tissue to be returned to the freedom of the outdoors to Stubby, who patiently lent herself to whatever my mood and situation needed.

After the chicken revelation, I could not stand to eat meat. And so began eight years of the "Meat War," with my parents wanting to show they were in control by placing five or so morsels of meat on my plate each night. As artfully as a preschooler could, I slipped my token pieces of meat to Stubby under the table. As the years went on, I became more sophisticated in my strategy for ridding my plate of meat, until finally at age twelve my meat-and-potatoes, German-descendant parents resigned themselves to having a daughter with strange eating habits, and they left me to my own eating routine.

Finding the Gifts in the Challenges

Sometimes I wonder what it would have been like if my parents had been tolerant or even supportive of my food choices. In truth, their attitude was completely consistent with their own upbringing and the views of that time period, and I don't blame them. That's just the way it was, and that's okay. Better than okay, really. There were gifts to be gotten. For example, I learned to rely on my own instincts and develop my own creative strategies to get what I felt called toward.

Whether we like to admit it or not, challenges and contrasting experiences are necessary for growth. The butterfly's wings are not strong enough to fly until she struggles to break the cocoon. Light doesn't exist without dark. We can't see the true brilliance of a star until it is outlined by darkness.

An interesting thing happens when you realize that there is a teaching moment in the challenge at hand. If you are open to it in the moment, there is the opportunity to gain insight into how to remedy the situation instantly. And if you are open to reflecting on the incident later, you may gain insight into how to change similar situations for the better. Sometimes it's as simple as admitting to yourself or another, "I'm sorry. I understand now." Yogi Bhajan had a saying that sums it up well for me: "Stand under in order to understand." When we stand under a situation, as Sarah did when she gave Kevin a yoga tool to help him help himself, we have the ability to see from a humble yet broader perspective. In the wake of that insight, solutions appear.

★★★

Can you think back on something that happened to you that you resisted, hated, or wished were different, and now you realize that you gained wisdom that you could not have if you hadn't had that experience? When you decide to change the way you see challenges, two things happen:

- First, you relieve yourself of the discomfort of the challenge.
- Second, you feel good, and that brings you into alignment with your authentic Self.

The Energy Between Us

As we move through the ideas in this book, the word *vibration* will be used on occasion. This word describes the energy between us, also known as the "energy of each moment." Every thought, every feeling, and every action has a particular frequency of energy, or vibration. The Free Dictionary defines vibration, in the sense that I am using it, as "a distinctive emotional aura experienced instinctively." I like the description of vibration as an "emotional aura," because I feel it accurately describes the tone of the frequency that we emanate at any moment. If I am sad, my emotional aura, or signal, is of the frequency of sadness. If I am happy, the signal I emit is joy. Others who come into my energy field pick up on that signal either consciously or unconsciously and respond to it. The really good news—and one of the main themes of this book—is that we can learn to become mindful of our vibration and, with practice, consciously choose the vibration we want to feel.

It is said that the great engineer Nikola Tesla once stated that "if you want to find the secrets of the universe, think in terms of energy, frequency, and vibration."

This atmosphere of thinking in terms of energy and vibration is the new luminous space we are feeling for in our relationship with ourselves and, in turn, with our children. Consider the following scenario and the various energy vibrations that it contains.

Mom (or Dad) is driving with a four-year-old who is sitting in a car seat in the back. They are driving down a highway when another car cuts them off, and Mom has to slam on the brakes to avoid an accident. Mom begins to swear, then tries to calm down. The child notices the dramatic change in her parent's energy. This child can tell that something upsetting has happened, so she asks, "What's the matter, Mom?"

Let's say Mom chooses to "protect" the child by saying, "Nothing, honey. Everything is fine." Then Mom looks at the small child through the rearview mirror, trying to smile, but her smile doesn't really reach her eyes because she's scared. The child, being intuitive about feelings, knows that something is not fine. So this one little incident becomes one of many little incidents for the child, and over time the child begins to believe that either (1) "adults do not tell the truth, because what they say does not match what I can feel, so they cannot always be trusted," or (2) "since adults are bigger and wiser and must be telling the truth, I must not be perceiving the situation correctly." This is how children begin to mistrust their own guidance.

Now, since every cloud has the proverbial silver lining, we can turn this scenario around so it becomes a gift. The same near-accident happens, but this time when the child says, "What's the matter, Mom?" Mom says, "That car cut me off and I got scared we'd have an accident, so I got a little upset. But everything is okay now. I am calming myself down by taking some deep breaths. Do you want to do this with me?" Then she glances at her child with an encouraging smile. Now the child can relax and feel safe. The child also gains three profound understandings:

1. "Things happen in life that I may get upset about."
2. "It is okay to admit that."
3. "There are tools, such as breathing, that I can use to help myself feel better on the spot and recover my connection to my inner self."

Obviously Mom or Dad or Teacher would do well to practice centering techniques such as breathing or meditation at times when there is a lull in the action. Centering practices set the stage for positive experiences when life with children presents the threat of a storm, and they can even help avoid a full-blown hurricane-level interaction.

Knowing that practice makes perfect, I have joined the ranks of many parents who have found greater motivation to stay on target since having a child. I use yoga, meditation, journaling, present moment awareness—whatever it takes! Nothing beats a consistent daily practice of whatever speaks to your soul and tunes up your awareness, be it yoga or a run on the beach. If you regularly touch and verify your inner connection to your authentic Self, you won't stray too far in your interactions with your child. Whether you're having trouble with your child or with your own life, the issue won't be so serious, and you won't take it so seriously. When difficulty arises, your attitude will be less "this is a big problem" and more "what can I learn from this?"

***

In my yoga path, we always take a moment to center ourselves with the breath or sound before starting a project. This is a great habit to get into, even for small things such as answering the phone mindfully, getting ready to drive a car, or having a conversation with your child. The centering makes all the difference in the interaction. In my Montessori training, we were told to get on the level of the child and look into their eyes with an open, supportive attitude. I think of this as answering an invitation into their world. In my many years of practice with this simple technique, I have always found that I can really feel the essence of the child, and our interaction is much richer and respectful. In slowing down and centering ourselves, we can be with just this moment, and this automatically accesses the intuitive mind. Albert Einstein's perspective on intuition, according to Bob Samples in his book *The Metaphoric Mind*, was that "the intuitive or metaphoric mind [is] a sacred gift ... the rational mind [is] a faithful servant. It is paradoxical that in the context of modern life we have begun to worship the servant and defile the divine." [2]

One of my students, a children's yoga teacher named Sari, wrote to me after taking the Radiant Child training. She experienced this "invitation" in this way: "Without a doubt the most important technique that I learned, and am now practicing, is watching my own energy 'signal' and what emotions I am bringing to class. The children are extremely sensitive to my energy and can truly pick up when I'm off-center. They also emit a special and pure energy that has changed me profoundly. I find myself more confident, radiant, and full after teaching them, when, in fact, I think that they are the ones who teach me! What I've found is a world of innocence, pure joy, and wonder. I see them in such a different light, and they have truly changed my life. I approach teaching them without a 'let's fix this' attitude, and I know and feel that they see me as a safe energy, where they can be themselves and we can explore together."

More and more parents and teachers are practicing the "highest yoga" by relating to children with an attitude of wholeness of body, mind, and spirit. Life becomes so interesting and, yes, even extraordinary once we start the inner journey toward being who we actually are, our authentic Selves. It's at this place that we sense what truly exists and find ways to deal with what life brings us in a more graceful, connected manner.

Fathering from the Soul: Kartar's Perspective

If the expression of deep peace throughout all the winds of change is your intention, you will begin to see it manifesting. One of the most deeply peaceful and steady-hearted people I know is Kartar, my husband. Without his wisdom and involvement, this book could not be complete. Also, without the valuable perspective of fathering from the yogic or soul level, we would be missing an amazing opportunity to

2. Quote Investigator, "The Intuitive Mind Is a Sacred Gift and the Rational Mind Is a Faithful Servant," http://quoteinvestigator.com/2013/09/18/intuitive-mind.

help better raise a conscious, soul-connected child. Because of the importance of all parental and adult roles, I want to take this opportunity to share something with you that comes from Kartar's loving heart and his wise perspective:

> One of the major anchor points that helped prepare me to father a child was the question that Yogi Bhajan asked Shakta and me: "Why do you want to have a child?" This was an important question and one that we both weighed heavily, each coming to our own independent answer. My answer was that I wanted to father a soul who would have such peace and clarity that he or she would be of great assistance to others. My feelings about this were clear, and I knew in my bones that this was what I wanted.
>
> When Ram Das was still very young, I would gather him up in a backpack and we'd go out for a walking meditation. I held the intention to let him be absorbed in the vibration of the mantra I was chanting and the peace and calm that it was establishing in my brain waves. Occasionally I would arrive home from work and find that he was out of sorts. My favorite thing to do was just to scoop him up and go for one of our walks. I thought of it as resetting the energy and coming back to center. The ability to reset and center is something he can still relate to, and though they may not take the same form as yoga and meditation, he has his own ways of regaining balance that work for him.
>
> In addition to the private walks I took with Ram Das, Shakta and I did hour-long walking meditations for many years. Our son came along in the backpack for hundreds of these. Sometimes there was talking, but many times we just used sound and the vibration of chanting to establish a pattern of deep peace.
>
> This place of deep peace is now "home" for Ram Das. I may never know the role that these walks played in establishing a connected place for him, but I feel he does. I see this as an observer, noticing his even-keeled approach to important conversations

and actions and the way he can easily see the big picture in a situation.

On the opposite side of "quiet and calming alertness" is meaningful conversation. An important aspect of my relationship with Ram Das included talking with him from a soul level. I did this before he was born and continued on through his stages of growth in life. I wanted to share with him the way life worked, as I understood it.

There was one particularly memorable time. It was during the winter and I was on duty, because he was learning not to nurse in the middle of the night. It was cold, but we were well bundled as we walked in the magical stillness of the nighttime air. He started out crying, and I waited patiently. Between his cries, I spoke to him through my thoughts and actions, never saying a word out loud, and creating a soul-to-soul connection.

I explained to him that it was natural to be upset when something he thought he needed for his wellbeing was no longer being provided, that this was something he would see in many other forms throughout his life. He would be learning the discipline of knowing that all was well as it was, and to let go of what he thought he needed. I acknowledged his confusion and fear, and in turn, he learned to understand.

Through my own awareness and acknowledgment of Ram Das as his own individual, the calming presence I maintained, and conversations that were conducted soul to soul, I found the cornerstones of fathering that came to me naturally, as they were a part of my soul. I am so thankful that I was able to slow down enough to listen to the subtle guidance of the universe. Anytime I need to, I can still call on this guidance to stabilize the father's prayer within me.

★★★

Being at Zero: A Practice

There are an infinite number of techniques and processes to bring you to a state of soul-to-soul connection with another human being, as described by Kartar in the previous story. Yoga, meditation, chanting, breathing, and journaling are among the most common transformative practices that will often feel like the right thing to do when you need a lift. And sometimes you may feel that you have to let go of tools and processes and just "be."

Have you ever felt the need to let go and get down to the most basic level of existence—being purely alive, with no technique or process? Beyond all methods of personal transformation, there is an expansive space of just being alive, experiencing yourself as alive in the present moment.

Many people experience present moment awareness as both grounding and elevating at the same time. In yoga, we call this meditative experience *shunia*, or being at zero. Being at zero means you are not reactive to situations, including those with your children. In the yoga teachings, there is an analogy that any number multiplied by zero is still zero, meaning that when you are at zero, nothing can bother you. You are able to stay centered amid chaos.

Let's go to zero now by focusing on the one action that keeps us alive: the breath. Slowly read out loud the practice called Breath as Sensation, which is presented in the following section. Let the communication come from your knowing self, your inner self. Allow time for the words to soften your resistance and settle in. Allow space for the feeling of the experience to rise.

Eventually you may want to record yourself guiding you into this practice and any other practices in this book. This will allow you to close your eyes and focus on the instruction without reading. In addition, receiving guidance from your own voice is a powerful tool to establish an enduring link to your inner guidance. If you have not experienced this yet, I believe you will find it to be quite healing and uplifting to hear your own voice—which carries your unique energy—lovingly speak to you.

Breath as Sensation: A Practice

Sit in a chair with your feet flat on the floor. Alternatively, sit cross-legged on the floor on a dense cushion or blanket. Relax your body, with the spine comfortably straight. Close your eyes. Find a "let go" feeling, such as a big whole-body sigh. Feel your mind relaxing. Imagine your head thoughts dropping down into your body. Feel the swirling thoughts sinking down like sand sinks in water. Let them drop down to your belly, legs, and feet … and into the earth. Without any effort, just notice the feelings or sensations that you experience as you are doing this.

Notice your breath without trying to regulate it in any way. Feel the expansion and contraction of the chest and belly. Begin to slow down the breath and deepen it. Again, feel the expansion and contraction of the chest and belly. Notice if there is mental chatter—for example, comparing the original breath with the deeper breath. Become aware of any feelings that you wish you weren't feeling or thoughts you're trying to stop, allowing these things to become expressions of this moment. As the wave of thought passes, turn your attention to experiencing the body during the breath. Continue to breathe deeply.

Feel as though you are an infant resting comfortably. Since you don't understand concepts such as "breathing" or "expansion" as an infant, tap into what the breath feels like without any concepts. Begin to notice the sensations that arise, flow, and change within you as you breathe. Feel as if the breath is breathing you, as if you are experiencing yourself not as a person but as a breathing machine. Notice how your breath is happening on its own, without any effort or attention from you.

If thoughts come up, allow the sensations of those thoughts to be present, without pushing them away or following them wherever they might lead. If you feel resistance to any part of this process, allow yourself to expand to feel the sensations that arise in response to the resistance. Include the sensations of resistance. Expand to allow all sensations experienced in this moment. Just for right now, allow yourself to know that each moment holds a new experience, an experience purely without concept.

Stay in this awareness for a few more moments. Then gently inhale…and exhale. Open your eyes and begin to move your body softly. You will find that you can feel a lingering sense of your experience that you can call on in your daily life, more and more, as you practice this technique.

Experiencing Pure Awareness: A Practice

What does it feel like to be purely alive, purely aware? An infant knows, though he or she cannot tell us about it. But we can find out for ourselves by imagining the sensations experienced by a newborn—sensation without analysis, judgment, or even conceptual labeling. Using our imagination and feeling for the space we are calling forth in the exercise are the keys to success in this experience. Our imagination is an important tool in creating internal change. We use our imagination throughout the entire day, though we are often not aware that we are doing so. When we think about how something feels or looks or we envision what we want to happen, we are using our imagination. So let your imagination work for you in this guided meditation:

You appear in this world in your natural state. You purely and simply *are*. There are no labels, no agendas. There are no concepts. There is only being. To attempt to describe this state of being is to fail; the feeling of it is all we can hope to touch upon.

This natural state feels like absolute aliveness, purely being from one moment to the next, without even the sense of "moment." It is what is often referred to as spirit.

For a few moments, allow yourself to imagine this state of being purely alive. You don't know what anything means. You experience everything for the first time. A touch is not a touch; it is a sensation that begins from the outside edges of you, and in a moment that feels too short to notice, a response waves through you and produces sensations—comfort or fear, pain or pleasure.

A touch can be either loving or rough. You will respond in exact accord with the energy of the touch, though you will not try to do anything. The touch and your response are partners in the flow of life. There is no judgment about the flow of life, since from the perspective of pure aliveness, it is all just happening—happening to you, through you, and from you.

You don't know all of this. You *are* the experience. You know only what you feel. Your sensations and the rising emotion become your guidance. You are energy in motion—emotion. You know yourself by the sensations you experience in response to what comes from outside of this "you" that you don't know you are.

Gently allow yourself to come back to being you as you are now, and notice how you feel. Take another minute or two with this transition. Stay in the flow of the experience as long as you like or as long as it is naturally there. Continue with the intention of perceiving yourself as pure awareness as often as you can in your regular life.

What might you discover about yourself and your relationship with children in the process of being purely and simply alive?

For Children: The Feather Breath

The Feather Breath technique is something that creates comfort and awareness, making it a wonderful technique for people of all ages but especially for children. To do this, you will need a few feathers from a craft store. Make sure the feathers stand straight and have a top stiff feather and fluffy side feathers. Hold the feather in one hand, with the other hand wrapped around it, thumbs side by side, so you create a holder for the feather.

Bring the hands up close to your face so you can see the feather move as you blow it. Softly blow a long, gentle breath to move the fluffy feathers. Blow a strong belly breath to knock over the top stiff feather. Experiment with these two breaths.

Ask the child which breath is long and which is short. Paying attention to subtle cues like this helps not only with focus but also with body awareness and mindfulness. Then, when your child has become more familiar with this exercise, you can introduce the idea that the two different breaths have different effects. You may ask the child which breath helps them to feel calm, peaceful, and quiet and which feels more energizing or awakening. Since this question brings the exercise to an even subtler level, give the child a longer time to notice how each breath makes them feel. Generally, the long, gentle breath with the fluffy feathers is calming and the short, blasting breath is energizing.

In our earlier example of Kevin blowing the feather, the strong, forceful breath matched his emotional needs better than the soft, slow breath did. So that technique was a better choice, allowing him to release pent-up frustrations. The long, gentle breath would be a good choice before going to bed or to release anxiety.

Chapter Highlights

Parents, caregivers, and educators know that it takes effort to be a figure in a child's life who provides them with a model of someone who is connected to their authentic Self. How do we make it all work and come together in a harmonious way? Here are some simple reminders that can be helpful:

- **Become aware of life force energy:** When we remember that this is what we are made of, it brings us to the most basic level of existence and away from all the stimuli in the world around us. Take a moment to breathe before you begin a new project or important conversation.

- **Our thoughts and attitudes create an energetic signal:** Children are very aware of everything happening around them and are sensitive to vibrational energy, which means that they can sense what your "feeling message" is.

- **Become the child:** It's both a beautiful experience and an educational one when you can become the child and see things from their perspective, being more in touch with their feelings and refreshing way of viewing life. Take some time to remember how you viewed life in an innocent, simple way when you were a child, or just get into the feeling of it by observing a child.

- **Challenges are gifts:** Every challenge is something that we can learn and grow from if we choose to. When you find the gift in the challenge, suddenly you are vibrating in a new place, a place with a bit more light and happiness. Children notice the change in your energy, and in the long run, they learn from your example.

- **Respond to children authentically:** When we say one thing and do another, we send conflicting messages to children, muddling the distinction between outward appearance and perceived truth. Responding to a child with honest, thoughtful communication anchors the child in their own authentic inner guidance.

- **The yogic life takes practice:** Being aware of when we are straying from the paths that help us connect to our authentic Self once again—or maintain that connection—is something that takes practice, through awareness and a loving commitment to ourselves.

- **Children learn what they live:** We cannot teach children to be what we are not willing to become ourselves. When we commit to our own inner growth, we automatically begin the process of helping children to maintain or recover their natural, radiant selves.

CHAPTER 3

Walking the Balance Beam

In gymnastics, the balance beam is a litmus test for focus; the gymnast fixates on "just this moment," seeking perfect coordination with each step. The gymnast must not lean too far one way or the other, but instead must stay at absolute center. To bring the gymnast analogy to our relationships with children, each of us is a gymnast, and the focused coordination of our inner attitude and outer behavior helps us stay balanced on another beam—the beam of energetic vibration. In day-to-day life, our thoughts and feelings are behind each interaction with children, regardless of whether we are actively interacting or just projecting a thought or feeling about a particular child. One could say that a child's response to us is often an energetic litmus test for knowing exactly where we stand. Even if the child is off-center, we can use the occasion to work with our own ability to stay connected to our authentic Self.

Light Energy

When we think of the word *radiance*, we think of light. Decades ago in our ashram community, I remember looking into the faces of the children and seeing that their eyes, skin, and smiles seemed to glow from inside them. Something about that touched my heart and awakened me to the divine child within. I noticed something remarkable. For seconds at a time, there was no separation between myself and the child before me. From the subtle changes in the child's expression or action, I could tell that he or she also felt the oneness between us. It was in the air—in the vibration pulsing between us.

Connected to this newfound awareness, I began to look for opportunities to be with the little ones. I led them into imaginative yoga stories and simple yet profound meditations. I took them for walks, stopping every few steps to examine a leaf or a bug. I wrapped the littlest ones in soft bundles and put them to sleep with soothing chants and blessing energy. In following the path that children opened for me, I became a Montessori teacher.

I started my own cozy school where preschoolers ages three to six started their day with yoga and explored their natural healing abilities through learning massage and energy work on each other. After years of immersion in the world of children, I came to the realization that sometimes my interaction with a child could result in an outpouring of love. At other times it became a lesson about staying present with something we both might want to run away from. What I have consistently found is that as long as I let them in, these authentic humans that we call children have the capacity to keep me truthful.

The training program I created is called Radiant Child because I find that these words best describe a child's bright presence. In referencing the word *radiance*, I find many more words that describe the energy of children: vigor, ardor, eagerness, vitality, exhilaration, spark, spirit, zeal. Yet sometimes children do not express these qualities. Either they have lost the spark or the spark has turned to wildfire. Like the rest of us humans, they can complain, whine, throw a fit, get in trouble, and just generally be as far away from their connection to their radiant, authentic selves as anyone. There were difficult days in my Montessori school when they weren't cooperating or they were fighting with each other or running around screaming. I would think, *What have I gotten myself into? How much longer can I take this?* As the first school year ended, I had serious doubts about whether I would be able to continue to be a Montessori teacher.

Logic and Respect

That summer, while in a bookstore, I was attracted to a particular title on the shelf called *How to Talk So Kids Will Listen & Listen So Kids Will Talk* by Adele Faber and Elaine Mazlish. This classic parenting book saved my Montessori career and gave me logical and respectful communication skills that have become habit for me now. For my own self-preservation and out of a desire to master the challenge, I dedicated myself to learning new ways of communicating that would honor both myself and the children in my care. I posted the summary pages from the book on the walls of my school so that I could remember new ways of responding to challenges that the children presented. I found that by describing the problem simply and neutrally, without blame, the children displayed a natural eagerness to help. For example, instead of saying what I might have heard in my own childhood: "Who spilled this water? Somebody better get over here and clean it up!" I reframed it using my newfound skills: "I see some spilled water. What this needs is a sponge and a bucket." Miraculously, those same hands that previously pointed fingers at each other now gathered sponges and buckets, coordinating the cleanup until it was finished. I came to realize that when I communicated my respect toward the children, giving them a chance to self-correct, they responded to me (and one another) in ways that were worthy of respect. They tossed aside the blame game and helped clean up, even if it wasn't their mess.

From the idea of communicating with respect, another idea sprouted, something I call "making a cooperation." I introduced this concept casually, and there was never a lack of opportunities to practice cooperative communication skills in my little classroom! Let me give you an example, a scenario that actually happened in my classroom.

Imagine this scene: Two children, whom I'll call Josh and Bryan, are in a disagreement over playing with a toy truck in the sandbox at recess time. I choose to bring this issue to circle time so that all the children can have the opportunity to absorb the lesson as well as participate in the solution. Josh and Bryan come to the center of the circle with the truck. "Josh," I say with a friendly attitude, "how can you ask Bryan for that truck in a cooperative way?" Josh is likely to look into Bryan's eyes and respond with something like, "Bryan, I want to play with that. Can I have it?"

From there, Bryan may need some help with using honoring words, which is where I step in and offer this suggestion: "I'll be finished in a few minutes. Do you want this truck for now, Josh?" Then Bryan will hand another truck to Josh. It's at this time that I will continue to help the conversation deliver the best outcome. I may need to prompt Josh with an encouraging smile that speaks of how good cooperation feels. And then Josh responds with, "Okay, but I want that truck when you are done, okay?" Bryan acknowledges this, and then the two boys smile at each other. And another successful classroom cooperation is made!

In the circle setting, all the children get to see how this works, and it provides them with a concept they can use in their own lives from that point onward. In my Montessori environment, this strategy was highly successful and it helped to create good communication habits that, in some cases, made their way into the homes of the children as they modeled cooperative communication skills for their parents to learn!

There will be times when children come up with their own perfect solutions, with no adult interaction required. For instance, Bryan and Josh might decide that it would be fun to switch trucks and play together. In any case, then as now, I have always felt that I was planting and watering "honoring seeds" in each child I've had the pleasure to know. And, in the bigger picture, all this lovely work is nourishing my vision to help create a more peaceful world, one child at a time.

Tending to Our Tendencies

There were always ups and downs in that little classroom of mine. During those intensive first years, I often wondered, *if children are close to*

Source energy, or God, when they come into life, why would they express any-thing else? At some point my question got answered, as I realize now that a child's soul is no different from an adult soul, that souls are souls, whether they are young or old. We all come into life with our own agendas, or karma. These agendas might be gifts and they might be challenges, or they might be gifts and challenges all rolled into one. On one hand, someone may be stubborn and willful. On the other hand, because of this willful trait, the person may be more self-determined and not easily swayed by others. This can certainly be a positive trait. For example, if a young person is self-determined, peer pressure to use drugs or other harmful substances may not influence that person. So a challenge can also be a gift when it is in balance.

We all come into life with gifts and challenges. In Eastern teachings, the way we use our attributes determines our karma. The concept of karma, from Sanskrit, literally means "action." It is the law that brings the results of actions back to the person performing them. What you put out you get back. As you sow, so shall you reap. That's karma. One way of thinking about this is that we all come here to work with—or play with, if you prefer—our karma. This means we are here to learn something or grow into something or find our joy through something challenging. Karma is neither good nor bad; it just is what we make of it.

***

We can think of karma as our tendencies and what we do with them in real life. I know that I have a tendency to be emotionally expressive, both negatively and positively, while Kartar tends to retreat into his "cave" to work out challenges in silence. This can lead to situations where we become critical of each other for our different ways. Yet at other times we can appreciate our differences and find a balance. For example, when life calls for balance, I am always learning be a little more like Kartar, and in turn, he also learns to be a little more like me.

Parenting Karma

Just as we come into life with karma, we come into parenting or teaching not with a clean slate, but with our own beliefs about children:

- Who we believe children are
- What we believe children need to know
- How we believe we should deal with challenges that children encounter

When we look objectively at ourselves, we can usually see how we have developed tendencies toward children based on our beliefs about them that mirror our beliefs about ourselves. If we loved to read book after book as a child, then we believe that our children should naturally draw from our enthusiasm and love to do the same thing. If we never cried when we scraped our knee, then we do not understand why our children do. These are a few examples of seemingly small things that create certain expectations we have for children. When they don't live up to these expectations, we find that we have created conflicts within us that don't actually have anything to do with the children. Basically, it's us, not them.

For the sake of clarity, I'm going to give you some general categories and observations about types of parenting styles and philosophies for the express purpose of helping you identify and clarify your own tendencies. These styles are not meant to be analyzed or worried about, but are given so that you can notice them and even thank them for showing you something that is good to know. An insightful phrase that has been helpful to me is "you can't change what you don't own." This means that you have to recognize a tendency and why it is there before you can move toward a new way of being. And don't forget that while I use the word *parent* here, these categories of parenting styles and philosophies apply not only to parents but also to those of us who work with children:

- The restrictive parent
- The indulgent parent
- Underparenting
- Overparenting

***

There are always going to be times when we get out of balance in our approach to children. For example, whether we are parents or teachers, our tendencies with children can lean over into the *restrictive* side or the *indulgent* side. Some of us are consistently one way or the other, and some of us can go both ways depending on our mood or the circumstance. When the restrictive side is dominant, the result is a mindset that is aligned with this philosophy: "Children come into life untamed. They need discipline and regulation, and they need to obey. I am the boss."

One mother whom I've named Donna knew what it was like to play the parenting role of the disciplinarian, though it was not what she wanted in her heart. Like most of us, she just didn't know what else to do. I met Donna when she participated in one of my workshops.

It was her first day of Radiant Child Yoga training, and she went home feeling so excited about the kid's yoga postures, breathing exercises, and games she learned that day. Even more exciting, she found that she had a new perspective on her challenge trying to get Jennie, her six-year-old daughter, to do her homework each day. Jennie, who was in first grade, had a history of difficulty with writing the letters of the alphabet. Because it was so challenging for her, Jennie's morale was low, and each day she expressed a lot of resistance when it came to homework time. When I asked Donna how she would describe Jennie in regard to doing homework, she responded with "shut down." This resulted in both mother and daughter having developed a pattern of feeling frustration and some anger toward each other on a daily basis.

Donna left the course that day feeling that she had some new tools and was excited for the possibility that something new could happen with this situation, but when she arrived at home, she found a familiar scene: Jennie was at the kitchen table with her homework, struggling with writing. This time it was the letter *g*. Within a short amount of time, Jennie felt so frustrated in her attempt at writing that she threw down the pencil and paper, ran into her bedroom, and curled up in a ball on the bed. Donna's heart was heavy. She didn't want to go into the room and talk down to her daughter, forcing her to do the work, as she would have done just the day before. After the workshop, she wanted to honor and connect with her daughter in an authentic way. Donna recalled how she had felt when her mother tried to force her to do difficult homework, and she didn't want to repeat that pattern with her own child. She wanted something new to happen.

In Jennie's bedroom, Donna tried to get her daughter to look up at her, but she wouldn't. She asked again, but still nothing changed. Just as Donna was about to start in on the usual power play, she realized how much this situation was hurting her. She really didn't want to pass on to her daughter the way she had been brought up. It created this intense sadness, and Donna felt desperate as she realized that she needed to breathe to let some of it out. Suddenly she remembered a breathing technique she had learned that day called Balloon Breath. "Hey, Jennie, breathe with me. Come on! Fill your balloon up with air!" Then Donna inhaled deeply and raised her arms up as if she were making a circle, and then brought her arms down as she blew out the breath. According to Donna, "Jennie thought I had gone a bit crazy, but she did bring her arms up halfheartedly and breathe."

When she was done with this exercise, Donna felt a little better and thought her daughter didn't look as defeated as she had previously. She felt encouraged to introduce another yoga tool that she had learned that same day. Playfully coaxing Jennie into joining her in Downward Dog for starters, Donna then went into a yoga movement called Bear Walk. She began walking around the room and growling like a bear to release anger and frustration, and she encouraged Jennie to do the same, telling her, "Come on! Get out that frustration! Really growl like you mean it!"

Soon they were both smiling and even laughing at themselves. Donna felt lighter in her chest, sensing the heaviness dissipating in herself and in Jennie. At the end of the playful yoga session, Donna and Jennie sat down on the bed. Without much talking, Jennie picked up the paper and pen and did her homework faster than Donna had ever seen her do it. Donna didn't interfere. She just felt grateful that she'd learned some techniques that worked and that she'd had the intuition to use them.

Donna's story is a good example of how we can recognize when we are being too strict. When we replace our old patterns with a sincere desire to lighten up, we can see how there's room for new ideas and new creativity.

On the other side of the scale, we have the indulgent parent, whose mindset is something like this: "Children are perfect if you leave them alone. They should be allowed to do whatever they feel like doing. I am here to give them what they want. I am the servant." We've all seen this parent and child in a restaurant, usually at the table right next to us! The child is whining and running around the table. The child screams if the parent tries to corral him, and really causes a scene. Then it gets more interesting: the parent begins begging or bribing the child. This is clearly not a one-time situation, because the parent is at a loss for what to do—the parent is under the command of the child. You wonder, *how did that happen?* Or you think, *I would never let that happen!*

I've met, and even been, this kind of parent and teacher on occasion. Once, I was teaching a series of children's yoga classes to six- to nine-year-olds in an after-school club. The after-school teacher was of the "got to keep them in line" philosophy. In one class she pointed directly at one eight-year-old boy and said, "If that one gives you trouble, just let me know. He'll have to sit and just watch."

After so many years of retraining myself to hold an honoring attitude toward children and to communicate with them in honoring ways, I am not proud to admit that I did feel judgmental toward the teacher for showing her restrictive side, especially since she was disrespecting one child in front of all the others. So without realizing it, I tipped the scale to the side of indulgence instead of following my usual playful and structured way of teaching. There was no "Remember to stay on your mat. This is your island and all around you is water." Or "Remember, we are breathing, not talking. When I give you a signal, we will all do Balloon Breath together, so watch for the signal." Instead, I made the class too playful and had no really clear boundaries. Soon the children were acting as if they were at a fun, wild birthday party, jumping around the room, wrestling each other, and definitely increasing the decibel level by one hundred percent. I actually was grateful when the teacher stepped in and brought some sanity back to the room with her booming "All right, everybody, stop! Go back to your mats and sit down." It was a humbling but good lesson in striking a balance by providing structure and focus first and then allowing for creativity and freedom within the boundaries of the structure.

Coupled with these two mindsets is another factor: underparenting or overparenting. Both restrictive and indulgent parents can either underparent or overparent. Underparenting often happens when parents feel overworked and are dealing with a lot of challenges in their own lives. They may be preoccupied with issues in their adult world—money or career matters, for example—that are consuming all their energy, so there's little left for what is happening in their kids' worlds. It's not that they don't love their children; it's just that there is only so much they feel they can handle in any given moment.

Other times, a parent is very self-involved and doesn't take the time to put energy into their child. Another type of underparenting can be found in the case where a parent doesn't understand how to be involved in their child's life in a proper way because they don't feel a natural connection to children. Whether out of fear or frustration, they slowly (and usually unknowingly) retreat into the "safer" adult world.

Conversely, overparenting can appear in the form of overprotecting—not giving children space to experience life, make choices, or think for themselves. Often this type of parent lives out their life through their children's lives. I've had a few parents like this in my children's yoga classes. Usually I ask all the parents to come back when the class is over, but occasionally I'll have a hovering parent who asks to stay and watch. It almost never works out well. The added element of having Mom or Dad watching changes the child's experience and divides the child's energy. Children need freedom to just be themselves and not be someone's child all the time.

Overparenting can also manifest as an intensively scheduled life for the parent and child, which is often the result of an overachieving attitude on the parent's part. This is a concern that will be addressed more fully later in the book when we discuss how our life's momentum impacts us as adults as well as our children. Honestly, most of us tend to overparent in certain areas, if not many areas. Some examples are school work, sports, children's activities, and forming peer groups. What we need to do is remember where balance exists and why it is necessary.

Now we have at least four variables that can be combined to create unique parenting styles. For example, one parent may be primarily restrictive and underparenting while the other is indulgent and overparenting. In either case, the key words are *under* and *over*, which indicate that something is out of balance. To put it in terms that are inspired by Robert Southey's childhood classic "Goldilocks and the Three Bears," balance is not too much and not too little … it is just right!

You can feel when it is "just right" because it feels good, feels true. Whether the imbalance is from overdoing or underdoing, neither feels good, so being in tune with the underlying feeling is the key to knowing where some inner work needs to be done and how to pivot yourself in the direction of a solution.

★★★

The Three Minds

Yogi Bhajan used to describe worrying as "praying for what you don't want." In other words, what you focus on increases. Our focus is like a beam of light or a beam of energy, so we want to focus the beam on where we want to go, not on what we perceive is going wrong. All throughout these pages, we'll be working with these ideas and using processes to move in the direction of where we want to go. So don't worry—your "beam" can shine on the idea of balance! You can vibrate on *solution* rather than *problem*. We'll work on it here together, using a yogic teaching called the Three Minds: the negative mind, the positive mind, and the neutral mind.

The negative mind always tells you what could go wrong, what is going wrong, and what will go wrong. Its purpose is to caution you and keep you safe. It serves the purpose of helping you know the boundaries and limitations of any situation or idea. When the negative mind goes overboard, you feel limited by your self-imposed restrictions. You don't know how to get to the solution because you don't see that the problem can be viewed as an opportunity to learn. When the negative mind is habitually in charge, you rain on your own parade and everyone else's too!

On the other hand, the positive mind always tells you what is good about whatever is happening, what the potential is in the situation. Its purpose is to lead you into new ways of thinking and feeling and help you move into new areas of interest. With the positive mind in charge, you see opportunities where others may see problems. You are using the positive mind well when you see the gift in a challenge. But just as the negative mind can become exaggerated, so can the positive mind. When the positive mind is not in balance, you become gullible and overly optimistic. You don't have foresight or a plan of action, and you may find yourself entangled in challenging situations because you were naive and didn't consult the cautionary negative mind.

Enter the neutral mind. The neutral mind is not *in between* the negative mind and the positive mind; it is *above* them. Think of an equilateral triangle, with negative and positive angles at the base and the neutral mind forming the peak. The neutral mind takes the bird's-eye view of the situation; it sifts through the negative and positive viewpoints and mines out the jewels that they have to offer. Then, from the panoramic perspective, the neutral mind intuits the direction to take. The neutral mind is intuitive and automatic. Another little saying of Yogi Bhajan's is that "your neutral mind will give you the answer within nine seconds." Solutions come from the spontaneous insights of the neutral mind.

★★★

Let's take another look at the situation where the children in my school were learning to cooperate.

- The neutral mind came up with the solution by honoring the negative mind, which said: "I want the truck." "I'm using it."
- The positive mind was recognized: "We are going to create a cooperation. We know we can do it."
- And from that honoring, the neutral mind was able to see the natural solution: "Because honoring one another is the most important thing we are doing, a solution rises up naturally."

The Compassion of the Neutral Mind

Honoring ourselves and one another is a big lesson that we are all learning, and coming to neutrality is one powerful way to get there. Cristin is a Kundalini Yoga teacher and a trainer for Radiant Child who has used the negative, positive, and neutral minds concept for many years and feels it is of great value to her peace of mind. She is a dynamic, aware, take-charge kind of person who is married to a wonderful man who grew up in a different culture and has a personality that is very different from Cristin's. Her husband is fairly quiet and has a more laid-back approach to life and to parenting their children as well. They have a very sensitive, super-smart seven-year-old daughter and two tumbling, energetic three-year-old twin boys who love to copy their big sister.

Shifting from parenting a girl to boys and from one to three children has required a lot from the couple. There are days when Cristin feels that she and her husband are not parenting in a manner that will best model the values they truly want for their children. Quite often, she feels that she is tough on herself or her husband, and when that happens, she is not calm and patient like she wants to be. When this feeling comes upon her, she senses that she is pulling away from being a team with her husband. Fortunately, at those times, her awareness of the negative, positive, and neutral minds kicks in and helps her. Instead of feeling overwhelmed, she notices the limiting thoughts, which then opens the possibility for a different conversation, first with herself and then with her husband and children. In Cristin's words:

> It helps immensely to look at my own thoughts through the three lenses. My negative mind says that I don't know enough, my children may hate me as they get older, 90 percent of this day was not how it should have been, we are not a team, and my husband is not parenting like me due to his lack of _____ (and here, I can name the problem in my loud, judgmental voice: experience, feelings, reading about parenting, willingness to try, etc.). My positive mind says that I know everything about parenting, that my husband will someday do what I suggest, implying that I am right, or he will at least communicate more and suggest a different way that we can try, and then we will learn to work together better. Even if that doesn't happen, our kids are pure Source energy and chose us, so if we are terrible at parenting, they will still be fine. Can you see how thoughts in both the negative and positive minds both help *and* hinder?
>
> Then comes the neutral mind, thank goodness! My neutral mind says, "Tune in, *breathe*, and do your best. You know more than you think, and parenting is not about doing but being." Both of us come from a place of love with our children, despite those moments when things don't flow. This moment on earth is not about me but much more—it is about gratitude for all of it: the children's souls choosing us as parents, the gift of all five of us, feeling that our paths have crossed in this cosmic way, know-

ing that we will all learn, grow, and evolve together. Also, my neutral mind tells me to honor all that I do, both what I am seeing as failures and what I am seeing as successes; to have compassion for myself; to give my husband empathy and space; and to live in gratitude for it all. My neutral mind reminds me to worry less and to spend more time focusing on self-care, especially my own health and yoga practice. If I listen to the wisdom of my neutral mind, I practice awareness. I breathe, recreating myself in each mindful moment. Then I can enjoy my family more and see the whole situation with awe at the magic of it all.

Practice: Sa Ta Na Ma Meditation

We can see how valuable it is to take the broader perspective of the neutral mind while honoring the positive and negative minds for the roles they play in our lives. How can we develop ourselves to more effortlessly enter into the neutral mind? One very good way is to practice the Sa Ta Na Ma meditation. In Kundalini Yoga, there are a few hundred meditations, but Sa Ta Na Ma reigns supreme as the best all-purpose meditation. Children love it, too.

Sa Ta Na Ma can become your mind's best friend. It balances the negative, positive, and neutral minds and is particularly effective upon waking in the morning or before going to bed at night. Plus, this meditation is great for adults and children alike because it clears the mind of old stuff—and that's why in children's yoga we've labeled it "the garbage truck"!

In the yoga tradition, using a sound in meditation is called a mantra. Sa Ta Na Ma uses the individual sounds that are found in the mantra *Sat Nam*, which means "I am my authentic (truth) Self." In Sa Ta Na Ma, the *a* in each syllable is pronounced like "ah." Each syllable is a sound vibration with a specific meaning: Sa—the universe, totality; Ta—life, creation; Na—death, dissolution; and Ma—rebirth, regeneration.

Sa Ta Na Ma uses several types of meditation tools together, including voice, mouth movements, mental focus, and hand movements.

- **Voice:** There are three "voices" used in this meditation. They are the human voice (chanting out loud), the voice of the beloved (whispering), and the inner voice (silent repetition of the mantra internally).

  The pattern of chanting this mantra begins with the human voice for two minutes, and then softens into the voice of the beloved for two minutes, followed by the silent inner voice for two minutes. Then the pattern reverses, so you chant silently for another two minutes, whisper for two, then come back to your out-loud voice for two.

- **Mouth movements:** During the chanting, your tongue may touch your upper palate, pressing the many meridian points that are known to be there based on the ancient teachings of acupressure. These movements stimulate certain configurations that activate higher brain functions and help to release unwanted mental patterns.

- **Mental focus:** Your eyes will be closed and will gaze gently upward toward the top of your head during this meditation. The initial sound (the consonant) of each part of the mantra comes in through the top of your head at the crown center, and the "ahh" sound flows out through your third-eye center at your forehead. You can visualize an L-shaped flow of energy, which moves in through the top of your head and out through your forehead. You are creating an "energy loop" as you repeat each part of the mantra. When you imagine the sound in this way, it strengthens the connection between the pineal and the pituitary glands.

- **Hand movements:** Yoga often uses hand postures, or mudras. In this meditation, you will press your thumb to each of your fingers (figure 3a) to form mudras. Coordinate the movement of your fingers with the mantra in the following way:

  1. As you chant *Sa*, press your thumb and index finger together.

2. As you chant *Ta*, press your thumb and middle finger together.

3. As you chant *Na*, press your thumb and ring finger together.

4. As you chant *Ma*, press your thumb and little finger together.

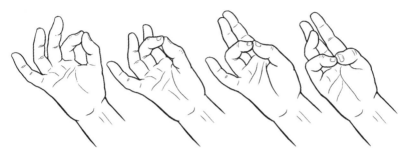

Figure 3a: Sa Ta Na Ma mudras

In pressing each finger firmly, sensitive acupressure points in the fingertips stimulate different centers of the brain for a whole-brain effect. This has been demonstrated in a study in which this meditation was practiced during a PET scan, lighting up different brain centers depending on which fingers were pressed.[3]

Some Suggestions for Beginners

As you can see, the Sa Ta Na Ma meditation involves doing a lot of things at once. I suggest that you begin by chanting the mantra out loud and then, when ready, add the hand movements. Then, when you feel ready, add the mental focus. When that feels coordinated, switch to whispering and then silence for a minute or so. Before too long, you will feel like you are in the flow of the meditation.

Here is how to set up for practice:

1. Sit in Easy Pose on the floor, using a pillow or blanket, if necessary, to straighten your lower spine. Alternatively, you may sit on

---

3. Aleezé Sattar Moss, PhD, et al., "Effects of an 8-Week Meditation Program on Mood and Anxiety in Patients with Memory Loss," *The Journal of Alternative and Complementary Medicine* 18, no. 1 (Jan. 2012): 48–53, www.ncbi.nlm.nih.gov/pubmed/22268968.

a straight-backed chair. Lift your breastbone and straighten your neck so your chin is level with the floor and slightly tucked. Place your hands on your knees, with your arms extended forward so your elbows are fairly straight. Close your eyes.

2. If you feel that it will help, use a stopwatch to do this meditation. Remember to press your fingers as you say the sounds. Keep visualizing the sound looping down from the top of your head and out through your forehead.

3. Continue in this way for twelve minutes, with each section being two minutes long. Inhale deeply and exhale. Then inhale and stretch your arms up high and shake your arms and spine for twenty to thirty seconds. Exhale and relax.

After your practice, take note of how you feel as you go about your day. Consider making it a goal to slowly increase the length of time that you do this meditation, up to a maximum of thirty minutes a day, with each section being five minutes long.

Children's Practice: Downdog and Bear Walk

Downdog: Kneel on the floor and then place the hands flat on the floor, right underneath your shoulders. Your back will be flat like a table. From here, raise yourself up so your bottom is the tallest point, like the top of a mountain. Stretch deeply in this position the way a dog does when it is stretching. Straighten your legs and push your heels toward the floor (figure 3b). Your head will be looking up at your belly. Breathe long and deep through your nose at least eight times, or more if you like.

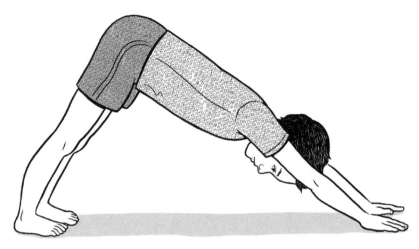

Figure 3b: Downdog

Parents, one thing that is wonderful about Downdog is that it is good for releasing tension and letting go of emotions that accumulate during the day. For an extra release, take several deep breaths, each with a strong exhalation using the appropriate sound of *woof!*

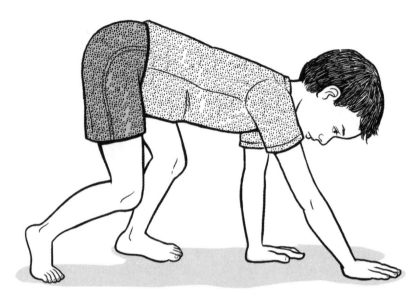

Figure 3c: Bear Walk

Bear Walk: Once in Downdog, begin walking. Ideally, you will reach out with one hand to the floor and follow up with the opposite foot; however, if the child cannot do this easily, allow them to do the exercise as they can. Begin walking all around the room like a bear (figure 3c). Keep your legs straight but not stiff, and allow your hips to move from side to side as you walk. Mimic a bear walking and make sure to growl! When you are ready to end, come back to your mat or your space and curl up in Child's Pose to hibernate. Breathe and dream a good bear dream!

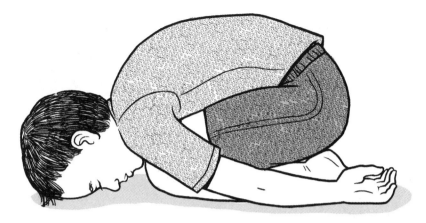

Figure 3d: Child's Pose

Child's Pose is done by sitting on the heels and then bringing the forehead to the floor. The arms are relaxed by the sides (figure 3d).

All these wonderful movements are also good for parents and teachers, not just children. Make sure you take advantage of the opportunity to connect with children through doing the poses with them—have some fun releasing your tensions as well.

Chapter Highlights

Most of us adults have had the pure joy of experiencing a magical moment with a child. It was a time when we felt a connection that stood out to us, whether it was a time when we were offering the child comfort, sharing a positive experience, or simply being there and letting the child know that everything would be okay, through our actions and internal thoughts. Moments like these can happen more often if we take the time to slow down and be more attuned to what balance truly feels like. Balance is a beautiful gift for a nurturer to model for a child. Balance comes to us as we become aware of where our vibrational energy lies. Toward that end, here are some helpful ideas:

- **Be proactive:** Notice what is happening in the environment around you that may be causing an imbalance or a struggle.

- **Make respectful interactions a habit:** Children are full-fledged beings who deserve respect and to have our full attention when they are in need. Since children learn what they live, parents and teachers have a golden opportunity to help them create a lifelong habit of respect.

- **Cooperation is a way of life:** Finding ways to cooperate that do not favor one child or person over another teaches important life lessons about handling conflict in ways that result in positivity, or win-win situations.

- **Be aware of your own presence and energy:** As adults, when we are in a bad mood, children can tell this and often feed off of the strongest energy we are relaying. Being aware of this is powerful knowledge that can inspire us to find our own balanced place, which, in turn, will guide children to their balanced place.

- **Not too much, not too little:** Know where your strengths and weaknesses lie, but stay in balance; don't overanalyze.

- **Let the three minds help you:** We have a positive mind, a negative mind, and a neutral mind. Think of a triangle, seeing the neutral mind on top. It is able to look at everything from a place that isn't emotionally charged but is aware of what exists at that moment. Ask yourself, *Am I vibrating on the idea of a solution or on the problem?*

CHAPTER 4
Into the High Heart

You are having a challenge with a child—your own or someone else's. You struggle with your choices: do you try to make peace or do you lay down the law? Then, out of nowhere and just in time, you experience an awakening of the heart, even if it is only momentary. In that precious moment, the fog of small-minded awareness lifts and you begin seeing and feeling clearly for a few moments, until the fog settles in again, perhaps less so. Remain with the encouraging feeling that stirs within your chest, and let your action flow from this place. You will know what to do because you have touched on your high heart.

On the journey of your authentic Self, you will touch on your high heart and have magical moments. Pay attention to these moments. Cultivate them. Remember them on your journey. And when those magical moments are in a dormant phase, learn how to use effort in an effortless way.

Directing Your Energy

In the beginning of the high heart journey, most of us have to make an effort to move in the direction in which we say we want to go. Even for those of us who have been transformed by life circumstances, an experience doesn't last forever, even a life-changing one. Eventually there comes a need to direct the energy through *effort,* which is not the same as force. When we want change, we must learn to direct our energy to move from a state of thinking by rote into an in-the-moment awareness. It's at this time that we can learn to relax in the moment, no matter what the moment looks like. This is the beginning of the process of moving into the high heart.

Take this scenario: Dad is in the grocery store with his three-year-old child in the cart. The child has a toy she plays with until the toy is no longer of interest. She wants to handle the produce and says so. Dad is absentmindedly picking up vegetables, putting them in the cart and mostly ignoring the child. Or perhaps Dad is saying, "Not right now. This is Daddy's job." Now the child is becoming more insistent and is starting to whine.

Something alerts Dad to what is happening, and he picks up on the cue that he needs to wake up and be present. He takes a big breath. It dawns on Dad that the child just wants to be an active participant. As Dad becomes aware of this truth, he is entering the high heart by coming out of small-minded living. He is feeling what his child is trying to communicate. So Dad thinks, *What would make this work out well for both of us? How can there be a cooperative effort between what I want and what my child wants?* With a smile, Dad can say, "Here is a bag. Point to the broccoli that we should take home and then you can put it in the bag." Now the child is happy because she is empowered to be part of the experience. While the child is busy bagging the broccoli, Dad can continue to shop. Everyone has the opportunity to experience grocery shopping from the high heart! And the next time they go grocery shopping, Dad can pave the road to cooperation by saying, "I'm happy to have your help. You can just communicate what you want straight—no need for whining."

It's easy to think of effort as exerting a force, but remember that when force is exerted, there is an equal and opposite reaction—in this case, it can be resistance or pushing back. Dad didn't force the child to sit in the cart and be quiet. He didn't force the child's attention to play with the toy longer than she was interested in doing so. He relaxed and allowed himself to realize that his child wanted to participate. And in that realization, the effort to control his child dissipated, and his effort to engage her was a natural response from the high heart. While this was going on, Dad was also laying the groundwork for cooperation, by letting his child know that he would respond to clear, neutral communication, not whining. These are examples of new ways of thinking about "effort." In cases such as this, the effort increases naturally, showing itself as a moment of power that comes with being alert and open to the high heart.

Many of us think of our heart as a physical object, but as anyone who has felt strong emotion can attest, it is much more than that. Leading-edge neuroscientific research has confirmed that not only is the heart intelligent, but it actually informs the brain. In her book *Playing in the Unified Field,* Carla Hannaford, PhD, explains:

> All the neurotransmitters found in the brain are also found in the heart. The heart actually appears to have its own sensitivity to the world, and exhibits that with intelligence, to the extent that the brain energetically revolves around the heart, and not the other way around. The heart generates an electromagnetic energy field (EMF) that is 60 times greater than the field of the brain (as measured externally by a SQUID).[4] It is the largest EMF within the body system, extending 8–16 feet around the body. People's hearts are powerful transmitters, constantly sending out light and electromagnetic wave fields. The physical "antennae" able to pick up these waves is the entire body with its sensory apparatus and huge heart field.[5]

---

4. A SQUID is a Superconducting Quantum Interference Device.

5. Carla Hannaford, PhD, *Playing in the Unified Field* (Salt Lake City, UT: Great River Books, 2010), pp. 58–59.

The Effortless Effort

Having a huge heart field really comes in handy when you tap into it in a stable and neutral way. This is what a friend of mine, Lisa, does in her public school pre-kindergarten class, which is in a low economic area. Some of the children are homeless or have a parent in jail. Others have a parent who is addicted to drugs, or the children were born addicted. Many of them have sensory integration challenges, ADHD, and autism. Lisa plays down her teacher role and plays up the role of the children as she tells of all the amazing things that happen in the magical environment of her classroom. She knows that her job is to make the effort of aligning with her high heart, and to trust the universal powers to do the rest.

For example, she had one four-year-old boy who came into the classroom with no speech. Little by little, he began to make sounds and a few words. On one particular day, he relaxed in the nap area with headphones over his ears and began singing along with one of the albums that I made for children. He sang, "I am brave! I am bold! My own spirit I can hold!" That must have been amazing to see! As he lay there, Lisa videotaped him singing and tapping out the rhythm on his belly.

She did not "try" to make him use words, sing, or move with rhythm. This came from him. Lisa's everyday intention is to see the classroom as a place where there is the opportunity for living in the high heart. Her vision is to create a luminous space where there is the possibility of knowing one's own power. Trust goes hand in hand with the creation of sacred space. Throughout all the trauma and drama that happens each day in the classroom, Lisa brings her focus back to trusting that the children know the way to their power, and she guides them to their own inner teacher.

Recognizing Moments of Power

We all have the ability to do what Lisa is doing, and we all do it at times. It is good to recognize those moments when we are in the flow or we are connecting with our high heart, because what we perceive will automatically increase. Shining the spotlight on what is going well gives more energy to the idea of things going well. These little day-to-day bright spots, when recognized, are moments of power. Recognizing moments of power as they are happening, or quickly after they have taken place, adds positive momentum to our life experiences. We begin seeing how we are carried forward into experiences that give us pleasure, and those experiences, in turn, give us the momentum to live in the flow of our high heart. As this happens, we begin to interpret all of our life experiences as blessings, because nothing is too much for us once we experience even a hint of what we are made of, which is love, light, truth, and joy. Why else would we humans come here equipped with a heart that has a magnetic field that is sixty times greater than that of the brain, a heart that constantly transmits waves of light into the environment?

Let's return for a moment to Lisa's classroom. From what I've seen of how she runs her class, it is clear that Lisa stays in her high heart as much as possible with these children. She knows that is what they need from her, and she benefits from seeing them live up to their full potential. The happy flow of energy can only happen in a space of safety, and Lisa understands this. This is not the safety of fenced-in rules and regulations, but the creation of safe space that comes from honoring the Self in oneself and each other, and from maintaining a consistent sense of order in the classroom. The children's heart energy flows back into the classroom as their spirits are nurtured. They flourish in surprising ways because this kind of safe space is infused with the electromagnetic waves of the heart.

Even district supervisors are sitting up and paying attention to Lisa's little classroom. At various times during her career, they have sent observers to understand how she is creating success that can be seen and measured. But the magic cannot be taught; it has to be caught by those who are ready to catch it!

Through these chapters, our work is to ready ourselves for the "catch" by clearing out the old patterns and raising our energy frequency. This can be done in an infinite number of creative ways, including those given in these pages. What a revelation it is to realize that life is just *this moment*, and that every point in time can be a moment of power when we perceive it as an opportunity to feel good and do good. Everyone—adults and children—are in a blessed process of learning what it means to live in their high heart, honoring themselves and each other.

Creating Heart Space

Through our deep and sensitive relationship to our energetic heart, we talk about living from our heart, giving from our heart, and our heart going out to someone. Still, it has been my observation that oftentimes we equate feeling our emotions with coming from the heart. Our heart encompasses our emotions, but it is not solely our emotions. The emotional heart feels love as personal—for example, love for my family and friends. Moving into the high heart includes and yet transcends the personal perspective, and is a gradual awakening of higher realms of energy that draw us toward the high heart space, in proportion to our receptivity to those subtle lines of energy.

My physical experience of the high heart is a subtle opening and warmth emanating from the upper chest. I feel it when I spend time with my own emotional sensitivities. I also feel it with my family, friends, students, and sometimes just someone I meet in passing. At times, the journey from the emotional heart to the high heart comes forward when I experience a touching story of loss or courage.

The high heart journey can initially be a crossing over from our usual thinking mode into the heart of the matter at hand. We then become aware of our feelings and allow them to be—even if the feelings are encased in pain and confusion. Yet I have consistently found that when I give myself permission to go into the emotional heart with the pure intent to understand and grow from the experience, I don't stay in the emotional heart, and I don't fly away in fright either. It is as if I tenderly pick up the essence of the fragile heart of the situation or the other person or myself. With sensitivity and empathy, I gather up the feeling of the poignant experience and fly into the crystal-clear sky, where I can see it from a bird's-eye view. As the witness-self who has a precious hold on her humanity, I see the pain and I understand it. What spontaneously follows is the opening of the shell to reveal the pearl within. From the elevated perspective that includes the precious human viewpoint, the shell is valued as much as the pearl. The high heart is felt. And from here, everything makes sense.

★★★

Looking at the plight of the children in Lisa's classroom, with their varied, but similar, stories of hardship, it is easy to fixate on the emotionality of their stories and feel sorry for them, to wish that their lives were different. I like to think that empathy helps us feel human with all of our potential intact, while sympathy drags everyone—sympathizers and the objects of sympathy alike—down into a hole that is hard to climb out of. Instead, when the emotional story surrenders to the point of view of life as a learning tool, there is transformation.

Who can know what each soul is learning? Perhaps a very adventurous and strong soul has decided to come into earthly life for the express purpose of experiencing victory out of extreme challenge. We cannot know. What we can do, however, is support the radiant spirit, the authentic Self, of each child or adult we meet. The high heart takes the high road, but it doesn't leave anyone behind. In the words of Carla Hannaford, PhD, biologist and educator, from her book *Playing in the Unified Field,* "When we see others in pain, or facing fierce challenges in their lives, empathy and compassion assist us to link with that part of our own humanity. But we can never know the actual function of those challenges or pain for that person. When we label someone less fortunate, we miss seeing his or her mastery and connectedness to the whole. When we tie into this empowered, responsible perspective the prefrontal cortex is more active, allowing us insight."[6]

---

6. Carla Hannaford, PhD, *Playing in the Unified Field*, p. 123.

One of the best ways to take the high road but not leave anyone behind is by seeing the gift in the challenge. Reflecting on your life, I'm sure you can see the challenges you've faced and how you have overcome many of them. Take some time to recognize what you have learned from being challenged and how the challenges have strengthened you or developed another part of you. Now think of a child you have been feeling sorry for. Perhaps this child comes from a broken home, never had a father, or has a mother who is addicted to drugs. Whatever the challenge may be, you feel your heart go out to this young person. The question to ask yourself is, which heart is going out to this person? Is it your "poor child" emotional heart? Is it your "this strong soul has taken on quite a challenge!" high heart? What I've noticed is that when I come from the feeling place of "this soul has taken on a challenge," I suddenly know how strong and confident this being must be to take on this challenge, especially early in life. I can feel the power and wisdom in the choice.

Acknowledging the power and wisdom in a choice is best described as an elevated perspective that is like a beam of light that radiates from one heart to another's. On this beam is a message of honor: "You know what you are doing. You are strong and worthy of the challenge. My love is with you as a reminder of who you really are." This is one of my most treasured ways of working with children, through energy communication. Anytime I go into this mode of being, I find that the children most definitely feel it and consistently respond positively, and I feel much better, too! For many years now, I've dedicated the "Long Time Sun" song (from chapter 1) to individuals I knew were going through major challenges. I can actually feel the blessing in the song going out as a wave of light and love to touch the life of a person in need.

★★★

Several years ago, I traveled to South Africa to train adults about children's yoga, and as part of my time there, I was invited to share children's yoga with caregivers in an orphanage. It was a bit overwhelming to see how many children there were, and to realize the potential they had for living healthy, happy lives, if only there was the vision for it.

At one point, I needed a baby for a yoga demonstration. Most were napping, and I was beginning to wonder if I needed a new teaching plan. At that moment, I found myself eye to eye with a petite five-month-old girl solemnly staring up at me from her crib. I lovingly picked her up and told her that we were going to show everyone how to connect with babies. Once in the demonstration room, with thirty pairs of eyes on us, I gently laid her down on the yoga mat and began gently massaging and stroking her legs and arms, feeling loving kindness toward her with every touch.

I spent some time engaging her with smiling, singing, touch, and movement. For the first few minutes, she turned her head away from me in fearful distrust. Her signal was clear, but I continued to draw her in with my vision of her as a precious soul here on earth for her own great purpose. I trusted my touch and my energetic vibration to soothe her fears and help awaken her to herself. And, as I always try to do, I remembered that the hand of the universe always co-creates with me.

Within a couple of minutes, she went from being stiff and fearful to allowing her body to relax. And from there, she became actively engaged with the process. She looked straight at me with curiosity and seemed to be thinking, "What strange and lovely things are you doing with me?"

A smile tugged at the corners of her mouth while I gently crossed her little arms, moving up, down, and side to side in rhythm with the yoga sounds of "Sa Ta Na Ma!" Finishing up, I massaged her feet, showing the caregivers how the pressure points on the feet connect to every part of the body. The entire demonstration lasted no more than eight minutes. By the end, she felt relaxed enough to fall into a peaceful sleep. I placed her in her crib, my hands and my heart warm with healing energy and appreciation for her and for all the dear children there. Spontaneously, I felt a prayerful intention release from my heart to the heavens on their behalf.

I may have felt the need to cry, as I know I did several times during that time in South Africa. When I feel strong emotions well up, I let them express fluidly. I know this is a natural response coming from an open heart. What I have noticed from years of present moment awareness, or mindfulness, is that nothing stays the same for long. The painful feelings that in the moment bring forth tears, even sobbing, have their life, and it is right to honor that life. Then, as the moments pass, the feelings subside. And something I've also discovered is this: the most powerful prayers ride on the intensity of the emotional heart combined with the broader perspective of the high heart. For me, this feels like a beautiful and authentic honoring of "what is," while asking the universe to bring more light, which guides us to a more enlightened outcome.

★★★

The "Wouldn't It Be Wonderful If" Game

Being with "what is" will help you ground yourself in the present. *Okay*, you may wonder, *so how do I move from being grounded in the present into a future that is heartful, uplifted, and authentic?* One fun way that really works for me is the "Wouldn't it be wonderful if" game. Sometimes I play this game by writing in my journal, or I may choose to speak out loud, and at other times I find that I simply work internally to change my thought patterns.

Here is how you play the game. Take a quiet moment to write this at the top of a piece of paper: *Wouldn't it be wonderful if …* Then allow thoughts to rise up—especially if they are difficult ones. Let yourself feel the unhappy thought, then turn your attention to the change you are longing for. Think of the situation as a coin: one side is the challenging perspective and the other side is the happy version of that same subject. You get to choose which side of the coin is facing up!

We all have moments when we have troublesome thoughts in our minds, either through our own mental patterns or from an external situation that we allowed to influence us. I recall a particular time when I was negatively impacted by an acquaintance who expressed disapproval about the way I was parenting my son. And I was in the same judgmental space—not agreeing with her parenting philosophy. Obviously we didn't see eye to eye, and it was distressing—until I remembered the "Wouldn't it be wonderful if" game. This is what I did. I wrote: *Wouldn't it be wonderful if I stayed closed to my own experience and lived life from there?* As I wrote this, I could feel how I was staying close to my life. It felt like my greater Self was helping me to switch my thinking patterns, and it felt so much better than being bothered by small, everyday occurrences.

From there I wrote: *Wouldn't it be wonderful if…*

- *I left others alone to live their lives? Like my friends, my husband, my son, even society?*
- *I found happiness in all the little things in life and let the bigger things take care of themselves?*
- *I made peace with all the different parts of myself?*
- *I cared enough about how I am spending each moment to make each moment worth living?*
- *my heart's desire for joy and inner connection became the dominant energy of me?*
- *I found a way to honor everything that happens and everyone it happens to, especially myself?*

By the time I wrote that last line, I was back to living in my high heart, radiant and smiling. So give this life-changing game a chance the next time you are in need of a reminder to let go of the small stuff and step into your radiant high heart. After a while, you will find that you don't even need to write anything down; you will be able to easily switch your thinking process to the positive side of the coin.

Loyal Friends: Breath and Imagination

How do we come to find ourselves in our high heart, our authentic Self, our energetic space of connection? There is no one way, but there are helpful tools and ideas. Moving from one state of mind to another, like moving from one home to another, requires a little help from your friends. When it comes to inner transformation, you have two loyal partners—your breath and your imagination—who are always ready and willing to help you move into a better space. When you feel that you are not where you'd like to be, whether it is in relation to your child, your partner, or a situation, you can call on your internal friends—breath and imagination.

Breathing is an interesting phenomenon. It can be done unconsciously or consciously. Yogic teachings encourage us to be aware of our breathing process and to deepen it for relaxation and release of stress. In yoga, the in-breath brings life energy, or *prana*. The out-breath releases spent energy, or *apana*. From a purely physical point of view, each inhalation delivers lifegiving oxygen to every cell of the body, while each exhalation releases waste in the form of carbon dioxide.

We can opt to use the mind's power of imagination to see and feel the dance of the in-breath and the out-breath. Using the imagination deliberately is one of the best-kept secrets in creating change in the body and mind. Consider the following experiment in the book *The Brain That Changes Itself* by Norman Doidge, MD:

Everything your "immaterial" mind imagines leaves material traces in the brain and in the body. Each thought alters the physical state of your brain connection. Each time you imagine moving your fingers across the keys to play the piano, you alter the tendrils in your living brain. From a neuroscientific point of view, imagining an act and doing it are not as different as they seem to be. Brain scans show that many of the same parts of the brain are activated in imagination as are in action.[7]

---

7. Norman Doidge, MD, *The Brain That Changes Itself* (New York: Penguin Books, 2007), p. 213.

Waves of Appreciation: A Practice

A powerful example of using breath and images, this next practice can be done anytime and anywhere—alone or in a crowd, while sitting in meditation or when you are in a challenging situation. It is a perfect practice to share with those you love because it grows the love between you.

1. The waves of breath flow up to the shore of your body on the in-breath. They flow out to the sea of energy surrounding you on the out-breath.

2. As the breath rolls inland, let it fill every corner and every pocket of your body and mind. Then let head thoughts drop down into the body on the first out-breath.

3. Breathe in again. Draw in fresh life, also called prana or qi. On the exhalation, let the head surrender to the heart as the waves surrender themselves back to the ocean.

4. Inhale. Allow thoughts of someone or something you love to enter your body and mind. As the breath rolls out again, feel your appreciation warming the heart.

5. Inhale again. Drop down into the heart, and grow the sense of appreciation. Let other thoughts and feelings of appreciation gather in the heart. Exhale and send your appreciation out to the world, to the universe.

6. Begin to breathe in and out through the heart center. Circulate waves of love up to the shore of your body-mind and send currents of appreciation back out to the vast sea of life.

7. Continue for as long as you like, and return to the experience as needed throughout the day.

Remember that a practice is just that—practice for real life. Befriend this practice, and it will come to your aid. You will be happily surprised at the ease with which these new practices will become natural for you. And, just as importantly, befriend yourself at all times, including times when you think you "should" have a practice but it is not coming easily. Remember that life is always a flow and a journey. To use the analogy of the ocean again, there are ebbs and flows to your life, so there will be ebbs and flows to your practice as well. You can get back in the flow much more easily if you allow for the ebbs.

Heart-Opening Relaxation: A Practice

During this practice, you may like to listen to a recording of yourself speaking the Waves of Appreciation practice just described, or you may prefer silence or soft music.

1. Lie down, face up, on a yoga mat, a futon mat, or a firm bed. Place a pillow under your knees for lower-spine comfort.

2. Using a bolster, a Thai yoga pillow, or a firm cylindrical pillow, place the pillow under your upper back around the shoulder blade area or a bit lower (figure 4a). Move the pillow around until it feels comfortable and is in the right place to gently open any tight areas of your upper back.

3. Breathe in from your belly to your upper chest, consciously feeling your intention to allow the upper back to open.

4. Exhale and let go of any feelings that may be hindering your freedom to simply *be*. Continue to breathe with mindfulness.

5. Feel your high heart opening like a door that opens to the light. Imagine your heart like a beautiful, small bird joyfully taking flight for the first time.

6. Let this vision resound within your body and mind with deep, conscious breaths, for as long as you like.

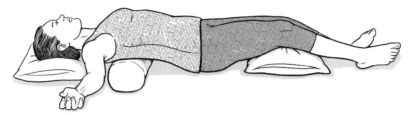

Figure 4a: Heart-Opening Relaxation

7. When you are finished with the relaxation, remove the bolster and draw your knees to your chest as a counter-stretch. Take several deep breaths, sending the breath into any remaining tight areas of the back or hips.

8. Rock side to side and up and down, then sit up. Notice how you feel.

Yoga in Motion: Children's Practice

Children love to sing and chant, which is fortunate since songs and chanting with rhythm activate both hemispheres of the brain, allowing for a balanced whole-brain effect. Children can either create their own movements or do those given here to accompany this positive affirmation chant. This practice may be done sitting or standing. Demonstrate slowly the first time, then repeat at least five times, up to as many as you like. Use this affirmation anytime there is a need to remember to be brave and strong.

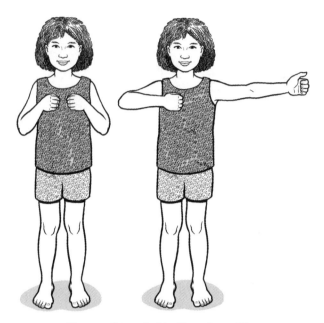

Figures 4b1 and 4b2: "I am brave!"

Say, "I am brave!" With hands in fists, tap your chest on the word *I* (figure 4b1). On *brave*, bring the arms into archer pose (figure 4b2). One arm extends out to the lateral side with hand closed. The other arm "pulls back the bow" across the chest with a grasping motion. The elbow is bent and and level with the extended arm. There is an open feeling in the chest.

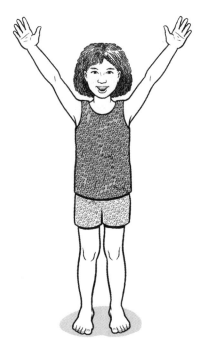

Figure 4c: "I am bold!"

Say, "I am bold!" Tap your chest on the word *I*. Push the arms up into the air and open the hands in a victory movement on the word *bold* (figure 4c).

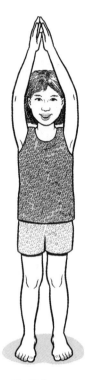

Figure 4d: "My own spirit"

Say, "My own spirit," and slowly bring the palms flat together over-head (figure 4d).

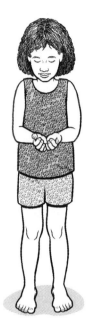

Figure 4e: "I can hold!"

Say, "I can hold!" Slowly bring the arms down to chest level and open the hands, looking inside them like you are holding something precious (figure 4e). And you are—it's your spirit!

Chapter Highlights

- **Learn to direct your energy:** Consciously make the effort to switch from a state of thinking by rote to an in-the-moment awareness. Then, by relaxing in the moment, no matter what it looks like, you begin the process of moving into the high heart.

- **Understand the high heart:** Our high heart includes our emotional heart but also transcends it. The high heart is felt from an elevated perspective, one that includes our human viewpoint. From this place, everything makes sense.

- **Acknowledge what science shows us about our hearts:** Hearts are powerful transmitters and are constantly sending out light and electromagnetic wave fields. When we are aware of this, we can make the "effortless effort" of directing our attention in loving, supportive ways to any adult or child we want to help.

- **Recognize our moments of power:** When we notice that we are connecting with our high heart, and we recognize these moments, they become moments of power. What we perceive will automatically increase. By shining the spotlight on what is going well, we give more energy to the idea of things going well.

- **Don't pity children with challenges:** Even though a child's challenges may seem so overwhelming that we want to feel pity, we can always choose a better path. Instead, focus on the strengths that a child has, as that will do much more to help that child. In this way, we can send an energetic blessing to the child, and even subtly remind them that they are a strong soul and can meet the challenge.

CHAPTER 5

No Place Like Home

We help children best by helping ourselves stay in alignment with our own inner being—our natural, authentic Self. Since this is who we really are, we don't have to make ourselves "better." When we bring it all back home to who we truly are, we uncover the being that has always been there. *We are who we were all along, but when we find our way back to our authentic Self, we return with the wisdom and experience that the living of life has imparted.* We are like Dorothy from the classic *Wizard of Oz* story, looking to find her way home and finally realizing that the ruby slippers on her feet were the means to take her home all along.

Many of us seek out experiences to make us happy or at least help us forget the hurts we may feel at times. We've all spent time looking outside of our true Self, searching to find fulfillment in achievement, recognition, material possessions, popularity, or any number of methods. We often lose sight of the fact that we already have all that we need to "come come" at any time, because our home is with us always; it's who we actually are. In other words, our ruby slippers are our authentic being.

It can be challenging to find a way to get back to being your Self. I want to share a simple, easy technique that I use: I "tune in" to children anytime I happen to be around them. I find children to be like little gurus; they remind me of what's important in life. It is fascinating to see life through their eyes. For example, when I am in a situation where children are making noise that my adult mind labels as disruptive, if I am aware of how I'm thinking about the situation, I can choose to change from the adult mind to the child's perspective. Suddenly I hear not a disruption, but a joyful enthusiasm for life. When I am traveling, I often will notice that I am rushing though the airport, mentally going through my checklist and making sure I am in control of my life. Once I remember to be present, I might still be moving quickly, but now I am also noticing a child with his hands pressed against the huge window, completely entranced by the massive airplane pulling up to the terminal. In front of me is another child. She is laughing with delight, skipping ahead of her parents and proudly dragging a small pink version of her parents' wheeled suitcase. Those tiny moments move me out of my grown-up serious self and bring me home to a place inside where I feel the wonder and delight of life. I like to savor these moments and let them influence my day. Reclaiming a fresh perspective is a secret transformational tool I use that comes from my best teachers—children.

In making the switch to noticing with appreciation, we end up thanking children for being an example of the wise, radiant Self. In a subtle way, we thank them for showing us our own essence and how to get back to our Source, to home. Why is this important? Well, besides the obvious benefit of feeling good in the moment, when we recognize the essence of the child, we now understand that they do not need as much input from us as we thought they did. That can be challenging to accept despite its truth. Upon further evaluation and going deeper into that understanding, we ourselves don't need as much input from others and society as we think we do either. Children help bring us back home to the essence of who we are, and as we all know, there is no place like home. Let this knowledge be your "in the moment" meditation, and let children show you the way back home to your inner guidance and naturally happy Self.

First, Make Friends with Yourself

Our inner home is built on the knowing that *there is only one relationship to attend to—the one between you and You,* your personal self and your greater, authentic Self. This understanding may be interpreted in many ways depending on your beliefs and your current mood. For example, if you are feeling disempowered in the moment, you may interpret the statement as though it is pointing a blaming finger at you. Your reaction will be to feel defensive, guilty, or hopeless. Alternatively, if you feel in a hopeful or uplifted space as you perceive the statement "The only relationship is between you and You," the experience can be one of relief, as you realize that your life and how it unfolds is all about you and no one else. And the best thing about it is that you get to choose how you view each moment. Realize that it is all up to you as to how you interpret everything that happens in your life. In the practice of that realization, you will empower yourself to move in a positive direction.

Whether you are feeling guilty, angry, hopeful, or totally blissful, befriending yourself, no matter what emotional state you find yourself in, is paramount to the process of inner growth. You see, when we befriend ourselves, we feel better, and that means we are closer to home, to our true Self. The change in how we feel also means that there is a change in our state of consciousness, our vibration. From an energetic point of view, befriending ourselves even a little changes our frequency, and tunes us into a world that looks a bit better. There is a subtle change in our relationships with children and everyone else; the feelings between us are a bit lighter, a bit brighter. It is the Law of Attraction in action, because what you put out, you get back.

As you do your inner energy work, you will be able to view life from your neutral mind and high heart. It will get easier for you to realize something that many people do not have an inkling of awareness about: that every other relationship you have acts as an in-the-moment mirror, showing you to what degree you are harmonizing your personal self with your authentic, wise, radiant Self. Remember, you cannot make the mirror smile, but when you smile into the mirror, it has no choice but to smile back at you, because the reality you perceive is a reflection of your thoughts, beliefs, and emotions.

***

A simple story demonstrates the mirror idea well. A friend of mine, Janette, was struggling to find the inner joy and acceptance that she needed to really embrace a better life after a divorce. Little by little, she came to have a real friendship with herself, one that transformed her relationship with her children and ex-husband as well.

Janette came to the realization that *everything* you want to change starts with making friends with yourself. Through a consistent focus on befriending herself, she learned forgiveness, which eventually helped her to let go of the self-righteous, negative story she had been telling herself for years. Janette had become visibly down on herself because she'd recently divorced. These feelings had lingered in her long before the divorce; however, they really surfaced in the face of this major life adjustment. Not only was she sad, hurt, and angry, but she was also concerned that the divorce would damage her children.

As she began truly forgiving herself, she found she was also forgiving her ex-husband. Slowly, through Janette's healing process, it became crystal clear how intertwined their relationship had been, each feeding off the reactions of the other. As months went on, she took the opportunity to dedicate her morning yoga and meditation practice to clearing out the old self-deprecating and fearful patterns she had been clinging to. This was her focus both in her daily spiritual practice and especially on the weekends when the children were with her ex-husband, as she had the time to really dedicate a good portion of her day to her inner transformation.

As Janette made coming home to her Self her highest priority, she became more stable in her inner alignment, and a wonderful thing began to occur—she found herself dropping the resentment she was carrying toward her kids' father. It became clear to her that the momentary venting of negative emotions did not heal the misery she felt underneath. Instead, it made things worse, creating distress in her children as they felt so acutely the division between Mom and Dad, the two people they loved most in the world. In fact, as time passed, the relationship between Janette and her husband improved to the degree that they both agreed not to disrespect each other, not only when interacting with the children, but in their communications with other people as well. Prior to the divorce, Janette didn't think this would ever be possible. Yet once she found the ability to love and forgive herself, coming to peace with the divorce was, in her words, "the natural result of going with the flow of acceptance."

Using many of the same tools we are using (yoga, meditation, mindfulness), Janette was consistently able to hold an inner conversation that blossomed into kindness and love for herself. Within one year, her attitude toward herself, her ex-husband, and her children had changed dramatically. She was no longer worried that the children were "damaged." Instead, she saw that they were fine as long as she was fine.

Marvelous things happen when you come back to knowing that you are worthy, that you are loved, and that you are your own best friend. Since the primary step in inner energy work is to make friends with yourself wherever you find yourself, the tools in this book can help you reclaim your natural birthright: loving yourself fully and being yourself fully as well. If you need evidence of this, you need look no further than at babies, toddlers, and preschoolers. They know how to be themselves perfectly because they are still "home." You might wonder, *What happens to us to bring us out of this state of connection?* It seems to me that at some point in early childhood, we began absorbing beliefs that were, for the most part, unknowingly impressed upon us by our families. In addition, we were inundated with spoken and unspoken "societal rules." We took on beliefs that were not naturally ours, and we likely didn't know we were doing that.

While I am not saying that it's not important for children to know the basic acceptable behaviors in life, our natural self already does know them, and lives them, without being monitored. So in our own child-hood, most of us were coerced into following the rules, and were found guilty when we did not. This is just the way life was and, to some degree, still is. But now, using the tools in this book and whatever other methods work for you, it is time to reclaim your love for yourself.

Sit in your home of Self, and find the wisdom in your heart to accept whatever qualities you might find. Acknowledge that you've taken on those beliefs from people who did not know any better themselves. As John O'Donohue, poet and philosopher, so eloquently states in his wonderful book *Anam Cara,* "You can never love another person unless you are equally involved in the beautiful but difficult spiritual work of learning to love yourself. There is within each of us, at the soul level, an enriching fountain of love. In other words, you do not have to go outside yourself to know what love is. This is not selfishness, and it is not narcissism; they are negative obsessions with the need to be loved. Rather this is the wellspring of love within the heart."[8]

Our Child-Self Is Love: A Practice

Compassion begins at home, with you. And how do you find self-compassion? If you are game for an interesting adventure, try this mirror experiment:

1. Stand in front of a mirror after you've spent some time in meditation or quiet contemplation. Look deep into your eyes.
2. Through the eyes, see the innocent, loving child that you were. Realize that you are still that essential being; it is your home base, and you carry it with you always.
3. Bring the feeling image of the child you were to the forefront of your thoughts and radiate it out from your eyes, celebrating that you have reclaimed your natural, radiant Self.

---

8. John O'Donohue, *Anam Cara* (New York: HarperCollins, 1997), p. 26.

4. Do this as often as you remember to. It is a wonderful way to empower your Self.

After a few years of doing this mirror work, the experience of seeing the wise and innocent child came quite naturally as I was interacting with others. For example, I might be talking with someone, and perhaps my mind begins to get a bit critical about what they are saying or doing. Suddenly, I will flash on seeing the person as a young child of three or four years. Immediately there is not an ounce of judgmental thinking left in me. It is totally wiped out the moment I see the person as their "child," because I am seeing them in their innocence and it brings me home to my Self, where there is nothing but love and acceptance. I invite you to try this practice, as I have found it to be truly magical!

Embracing Natural Cycles of Change

Many of us use yoga and meditation to improve the quality of our lives and the lives of our children. Still, I have never met a parent or teacher, including myself, who would say that life with children is perfect—nor do I believe it ever will be, or possibly is even meant to be! There will always be new challenges to keep us on our toes, but we can learn to meet each challenge with grace and success. We can also learn to see our personal evolution as a process of coming home to who we truly are. In the midst of confusion and chaos, we can make the choice to treat ourselves as kindly and gently as we would treat a toddler who is learning to walk.

I know this from experience. I recall a time period when my son made a transition in his relationship with me. It was between ages thirteen and fourteen. From my perception, he went from being a child who looked to me for a certain type of connection—a cozy and motherly type—to a young man who found that cozy, chummy connection with his circle of friends. To me, it seemed that I'd transitioned to the person on the periphery of his life, becoming someone he could come to for comfort and advice but who didn't figure into his life in a day-to-day way all that much.

In most families this transition is a gradual, almost imperceptible process, but our circumstances were different.

A little background is in order here. You see, Ram Das went to a boarding school in India for nine months of the year from age eight until he graduated at sixteen. This school was created as a place where children could study academics as well as grow in connection to their spirit, without the influence of the less-desirable effects of the public school system. Ram Das lived in a dorm with other children his age, many of whom he had known since he was born. Though they came from all over North America and around the world, annual community gatherings over a period of several decades had created an extended-family feeling from the time these children were toddlers onward. So in a very real sense, the children were like an extended family.

Of course, we missed our son deeply. Kartar and I could only allow him to go back year after year because we clearly saw how living independently from us was allowing him to grow in the most astounding ways. For example, he learned to work out difficulties with his roommates, bargain for the best price in the many little Indian shops, keep track of his personal things, and bear the consequences of what it meant to lose them. He learned that he could rely on himself and his own ingenuity to solve everyday problems and resolve complex confrontations.

When Ram Das came home in the summer, there was a great joy in the house. And when he returned in the fall, it took a while to go back to our childless routine. Yes, we stayed in touch, both with the parent-child connection that was intuitive and transcended time and place and also through phone calls and emails. And I almost always planned a trip to India for his spring break.

The year he was thirteen, I made my usual plans to go to India to visit. After roughly thirty hours of travel by airplane and train and bumpy rides in auto-rickshaws (three-wheeled motor scooters covered with metal sides and a roof), I arrived at the outskirts of the city of Amritsar, where the school was located. I asked around until I found his dorm room and knocked. The door jerked open, and by the surprised look on his face, it was obvious that Ram Das was taken aback at the sight of me. "Ma, what are you doing here?"

Now it was my turn to be stunned. "I—I came to visit. Your spring break, remember?" I stammered.

He recovered himself: "Oh, I thought you were coming tomorrow. Well…" And then he looked behind at his friends, stepped out of the dorm, and closed the door behind him. "Well, okay … I am just finishing something here. Give me a couple minutes."

He shut the door, leaving me standing alone in the hallway, silent and shaky, with a sinking feeling in my stomach. It was only a moment in time, but so impactful to me. When he came out, I asked if he was going to come stay with me at the guesthouse, like he did every year. "Um … no thanks, Mama," he said. He'd decided to stay at his dorm with his friends.

I went back to my room and cried because I knew that I no longer had a child. I also knew that it was okay that I didn't have a child, that what I had was a son who was a young man—his own person. Knowing and processing can be different, though. They certainly were for me, as it took about a week of grief—a week in which I rarely saw Ram Das. During that week, I let myself be present to all I was feeling, befriending myself without judgment. I mourned for the child who was no longer. All clarity gone, I was unsure of my role with the young man. And despite understanding what was happening, I still found that my life with him was turning upside down.

Grateful to be alone, I used the time wisely. I meditated. I breathed. I wrote in my journal. I walked dusty roads in silence. I talked to my husband long-distance. I let myself feel the space I was in. I came to accept it. I found that if I didn't hold on to the grief longer than it was naturally there, it would flow into another feeling, one that fostered an innate knowing. And that knowing was this: *he was doing what came naturally, just the same as the summer leaves turn to gold in the fall.* There was no shame in what he was doing, just as there was no shame in me allowing the natural process of loss to flow into a new awareness.

Remember my story (from chapter 2) of the mother in the car who was honest with herself and her child about her fear of getting in an accident, and how that helped transform the situation at hand? Well, this is my version…

After some time of processing the "loss" of my child, I enticed Ram Das to break away from his friends by inviting him to the only American-style pastry shop in town. As we sat and ate cinnamon rolls, I found myself honestly expressing what I was going through. Tears welled up as I explained how I had known him since before he knew himself—such a privilege that we parents have!—and that my mother's heart was having a hard time letting go of the child he had been. On the other hand, I knew it was all good and right that he was becoming himself, an individual. Even though he sank progressively deeper into his chair, uncomfortable at my display of emotion, I could tell by the energy between us that he was listening intently to every word I said. Eventually we went our separate ways, planning to meet up later in the evening. I felt some relief in my heart after this honest communication, and I hoped that he was able to really hear me in the highest way—soul to soul.

Later that evening, there was a momentous breakthrough. It was as though a luminous space had been created by the combination of the meditative practices I had turned to for help, my honesty and compassion with myself and with Ram Das, his ability to listen, and the trust we've always had between us.

We'd taken all twenty of his best friends out to Pizza Hut (yes, even in remote areas of India!). What a sight this was! Imagine twenty eleven-to fifteen-year-olds packed into two or three auto-rickshaws. There were kids hanging off the sides, scrambling up on the roofs, and crammed onto each other's laps. Everyone was caught up in a celebratory, fun-loving spirit, and the animated banter in the air was hilarious. I happened to catch Ram Das looking at me, eyes shining with intensity. Very quietly so only I could hear, he said, "See, Mama, you have lots of children."

I will never forget that moment. I felt tears rise up as the expression in his eyes and the depth of his words were instantly etched into my memory. The poignant message in that one sentence let me know that he clearly knew me from the soul level, and that his heart was reassuring me, essentially saying, "It's okay. I am growing up. But you will always have children—that is just who you are."

Somehow I had found it within me to allow the grieving process to run its course while working with it consciously. And as part of the flow, a deep honesty had been solidified between Ram Das and me. The result was an energetic space of soul-to-soul communication without the trappings of mother and son, and yet… that moment also lovingly embraced the roles we played for each other. From then onward, I had an underlying sense of peace with who he was becoming. The grief was no more.

Being Outranks Doing: A Practice

That's a simple story about letting go and letting a child grow into who he is becoming, and yet the turnaround was the result of *being* rather than *doing* anything. As much as we feel life is about action and results, the truth of it is that action arises from a state of mind and heart. In other words, *being* outranks and precedes *doing*. Remember the mirror image? It smiles when you smile; it frowns when you frown.

I've used some form of the following affirmative statements to guide me back home to my guidance before taking action. You may like to work with them by speaking softly to yourself anytime you need them. Try speaking these sentences in front of a mirror for a powerful and self-affirming experience:

I am willing to allow myself to be as I am.

I am willing to let my child be as she or he is.

I am willing to not know how to handle everything on the spot.

I am willing to let everyone have his or her own opinions.

I am willing to give myself time to grow and heal.

I am willing to give my child time to grow and heal.

As we can see from the previous stories, living consciously, or mindfully, takes practice. We have mental habits of constantly busying ourselves. Our brains are like computers with too many tabs open. It is good to inquire into yourself and ask, "Do I feel that I am worthy because of what I do?" If the answer leans toward "yes," just stop reading right now. Close your eyes and take a deep belly breath. Let it settle within you for a second and then exhale with a releasing sound of "whooo" or "haaah." Do this a few more times, until you feel something settle and relax within you. For this moment, we are going to focus on "just right now," so those mental tabs can close and you can breathe a sigh of relief.

★★★

The Only Opinion That Matters Is Yours

Being aware of others' opinions is within most of our natures; however, when we care too much about what others think, we temporarily lose our ability to be in touch with what is good and right for us and for our children. We find ourselves scurrying around trying to maintain a certain level of keeping up according to outside standards. It's time to take a moment to check in with ourselves and ask why we care so much about what others think. What does it indicate within us?

When you come from your true home of Self, you are neutral. You see that those who criticize are really criticizing themselves. You know that it is not about you, so you don't take it in a personal way. In that realization, you can be free of the burden of taking on other people's opinions. And because you are in your place of wholeness, where all is well, you can be generous of spirit toward them in your vibration, your words, and your smiles.

Another great "check-in" question is: *What is the point of what I'm doing?* Focusing on this will let you know if your actions or thoughts are honoring you and your children, or not. If the point is a fulfilling life and meaningful work, you can take inspiration from schoolteachers who have used Radiant Child Yoga training to augment the pressures of school life with yoga and mindfulness—many of the same tools that have been shared with you in this book.

A common challenge that schoolteachers face is that they would love to practice more of the yogic and inner work with their students, and they can really see the value of focus and calm in the classroom, but they feel overwhelmed by the responsibility to complete piles of paperwork and make sure the academic standards are met. Many of them have found creative ways to incorporate yoga, breath, and mindfulness into the school day—for example, having the children close their eyes and breathe with the ocean for a few minutes before a test. Some of the teachers have even made these tools part of the daily routine.

Based on the observations I've made over the past twenty years of working with teachers, the deciding factor in whether or not this intention becomes a reality is the teacher's attitudes and beliefs. Generally, the ones who are successful in introducing and maintaining this kind of inner work with the children have a strong connection to their inner "home" and believe their own guidance and creativity is more powerful than the system. Those who say it is impossible to work within the current educational system believe more strongly in the power of the system to squash any of their attempts at positive, innovative change.

The teachers who empower themselves do three things that we've been working with all along:

1. They address any important factors that arise from the negative and positive minds and then use the guidance of the far-seeing neutral mind. This brings them back home to their true Self.
2. They choose what they prefer without invalidating what they don't prefer.
3. They follow their bliss, which leads them to discover creative ways to execute the vision they have for their classroom.

Letting Go of Parental Agenda

Theo is a long-time yoga practitioner and the father of four girls between the ages of eight and seventeen. One of his strongest intentions is to honor his children's paths and not pressure them into a "parental agenda"; i.e., what he thinks they need or want, or should want. In his words, "I have always tried to see my daughters as friends that I am constantly getting to know as they grow up. As my kids grow and change, I find myself doing the same. To keep up with them, I have to evolve myself. Nothing inspires me toward internal growth as much as being a parent!"

Theo went on to say that in our society, part of "growing up" is learning to live outside the moment—making plans, acting them out, reviewing the outcomes, reevaluating, etc. The list just goes on and on! His way of staying in balance is to make room in his busy life to just be in the moment. Theo said, "In the ever-fresh Now moment, my daughters see me as a real person instead of a person with an agenda."

I asked Theo to share with us what he does when he notices that his parental agenda is spilling out onto his kids and he wishes to circumvent that course. He said he asks himself these four questions:

1. Is this what they need right now, or is there a better time to address this?

2. Is there a way to be an example to them instead of telling them what to do?

3. Who do they need me to be right now—an active teacher or a friendly listener?

4. Am I trying to make them into who I think they should be instead of helping them find themselves?

These are powerful questions, and when I asked Theo what happens after he answers them, he said, "I take a moment to breathe and just look at my daughters with fresh eyes. Often things look different after I shelve what I think needs to be done and instead make room to simply be with them as they are." We can all be inspired by this simple method that Theo uses to remind himself how to get off the "momentum machine" and instead be present to a joyful life with his children.

Getting Off the Momentum Machine

The pace of contemporary life has accelerated tremendously from what it used to be, seemingly growing more frenzied with each passing year. I see parents rushing their children off to classes, appointments, and social and sporting events, often one right after the other, with dinner in the car. Multitasking has become the acceptable norm. Parents and teachers alike feel pressured to keep up on the fast-paced treadmill of life's events. They're frantically attempting to maintain their footing on the momentum machine as the ground beneath their feet disappears as fast as it appeared.

What has this resulted in, really? It seems that many children are dragging behind or acting out in resistance to the pressure they feel from their parents and teachers, who are frustrated not only with the children but also quite often with the "system" of the momentum machine. In addition, parents and teachers are often fearful that the children will not "accomplish" whatever the prescribed goal is for them. Ironically, these energetic vibrations of frustration, anxiety, and fear translate directly into the hearts and minds of the very children they love and wish only the best for.

At times, I have been one of these parents, so I understand how time crunches and fast-paced living present themselves to us, despite our best efforts to avoid them. And, of course, we want to learn how to handle life when it is coming at us at warp speed and to model balance for our children.

Many times we ourselves are learning how to deal with life as it is, and as we do so, we become good models for our children. Other times we are given opportunities to examine our lives, and our children's lives, to see if all this pressure is really necessary. Toward that end, here are some questions to contemplate and journal about:

- Can I stop the momentum machine and get off or at least slow down and go at a pace I can enjoy?
- Can I reflect on what price I may be paying for this efficiency or this achievement?
- Can I stop in a moment of challenge and ask:
    - What is the cost of pressured living?
    - What is the cost in terms of my relationship to my child and to our family?
    - What are the long-term liabilities?
    - Is it more important that I get somewhere or do something on time, or is it more important that there is integrity in the connection I make with my child?

These questions never seem easy to answer; however, deep within us—and sometimes very close to the surface—we know the answers. They are logical to us, because they bring us home to our Self and, most especially, to our own children.

★★★

Imagine this scenario, which, if you are a parent or a teacher, is probably quite familiar: You are trying to get everyone into the car or the minivan so you can arrive on time for an event, with all people and paraphernalia intact. You may even think of this process as an exercise in efficiency. Suddenly the sensitive child, or the child who tends to "act out," begins to cry and scream. It's frustrating, but … can you see that the child is just acting as a barometer for the frantic energy that everyone is feeling? Can you come back to your inner home and find a compassionate solution from there? Can you review this scenario later in a neutral frame of mind and get some insight into how to handle this differently next time, or how to prevent it from happening?

Here is a simple tool that combines your imagination and inner wisdom to bring insight and potential solutions:

Imagine that you suddenly have the perspective of an eagle on a mountaintop. From this height, look down and see yourself in a challenging interaction with a child, possibly one that happens often. You may be quite wrapped up in the drama of the situation. You may feel that the situation is of paramount importance. Now step back into the eagle's perspective and ask yourself: *Is this issue really more important than long-term learning for myself and my child? In honoring and befriending myself and my child in this moment, what do I discover about this challenging situation?*

Through this exercise, we are likely to find that our issue stems from our desire for our children to do something that we perceive as *essential*, yet we lose our soul-to-soul connection with them if we push our agenda more and nurture our experience together less. What is being asked of us is that we find out what is really *essential*, and we can do that best from our inner home of Self.

A wise and beautiful book that I've treasured for years, *The Parent's Tao Te Ching* by William Martin, explores the theme of what is truly essential in raising children in asking, "Do you have agendas for your children that are more important than the children themselves?"[9]

Staying Close to Home

Many families are choosing to get off the momentum machine and carve out a homey feeling for themselves and their children. Desiree, along with her husband, Zeke, have created and maintained their vision of living

---

9. From *The Parent's Tao Te Ching: Ancient Advice for Modern Parents* by William Martin, copyright © 1999. Reprinted by permission of Da Capo Press, a member of The Perseus Books Group.

close to the land, away from the manic pace of city life. They live with their three children in the magnificent Sierra Mountains in California, immersed in the natural beauty of the mountains and valleys, alongside their animal companions—cats, dogs, horses, and rabbits. Since Desiree is a yoga teacher for adults and children, she finds creative ways to practice yogic techniques with her homeschooled children. I've seen photos of her children doing "bunny meditation," where each child holds a baby rabbit in their hands as quietly as they can, with eyes closed and hands in laps. They feel the breath and heartbeat of the bunny and breathe slowly to project a calm, safe feeling toward the little creature.

This simple yet powerful meditation is just one of many creative ways that Desiree has found to help her children learn life lessons, staying close to their home base, both in spirit and in the natural environment. Desiree recounts a very special experience she had with her youngest daughter, Amiliana, who was six at the time. While they were driving down the road, her daughter was sitting in the back seat with her friend and her brother. They passed by green grass, grazing cows, and the snow-capped mountain range as they were chatting away in their car seats. What Desiree began to hear was fascinating, so she pulled over so she could record it. Amiliana said, "When I was a baby, I wasn't smart like other babies. I did things from my heart, not my head." As Desiree shared this, it was easy to see why this would be such a profound statement and point of curiosity for her as a parent.

As the conversation continued, Desiree confirmed that Amiliana still thinks from her heart, not her head. You see, back when Amiliana was in first grade, after just three weeks of school, she was able to articulate, just enough, that she knew she couldn't spend six hours a day there and still be able to be herself. Desiree and Zeke had listened to that, and as a result, they decided that homeschooling was a better option for Amiliana and her older brother, Xavi.

According to Desiree, "In our homeschool system, Amiliana is presently a leader for an outdoor preschool where they sing, connect with nature, and learn from the plants and animals. She is a mentor for how to track animals, identify scat, build outdoor shelters, and choose edible plants. She rides trained mustangs and works with ponies and donkeys. When she gets feelings about things, we encourage her to listen. Although the state educational system may disagree, we believe that her intuition is as important to develop as her alphabet and writing skills."

Understanding that Amiliana is a highly attuned child has played out in interesting ways on several occasions. One time in particular stood out to Desiree. She shared that when Amiliana was five, she was riding one of the horses with a trainer when the trainer told her to go over a bridge. Amiliana said that the horse didn't want to go. Although the horse wasn't showing signs of hesitation, she refused to give the command. She sensed that this was the right decision, and while she couldn't relay it to the trainer, she stood firm. Later that day, Desiree rode that same horse and sensed that the horse definitely had a fear of the bridge. It was a situation that needed a stronger rider to work through. Desiree said, "I am thankful for her strong sense of intuition because it kept her safe in that situation, and does in her life as well."

Mindful Moments

Most of us wish we could access our home base, or our intuition, in the moment, as Amiliana was naturally able to do. Finding that connection in the moment can be challenging. Here is a simple two-step process that can make it easier:

1. Take a few deep breaths to calm your heart while relaxing your mind and body just a bit more.

2. Bring your attention to the immediate experience of what is happening in the present, allowing all the sensations it holds to be acknowledged. By doing this, you are practicing self-awareness, or mindfulness. Through mindfulness, you may find the present moment to be characterized by curiosity, openness, and acceptance.

Through these two steps, you can come into a state of mindfulness, and the benefits of the experience will be so much greater. A mindful moment slows down your mind and allows you to be aware of subtle nuances. It's similar to how a scene may be filmed in slow motion so the viewer can witness the subtle changes of expression on the faces of the actors. Slowing down and becoming mindful can lead into an artful and conscious directing of your thoughts and feelings, so your quality and enjoyment of life improves exponentially.

Try breathing consciously as often as you can remember to. Sit with a piece of fruit in your hands and feel the miracle of its creation from a tiny seed planted in the earth. Then savor each tasty bite. Find simple ways of slowing down and noticing life before it passes. When you are taking a walk, use all of your senses to appreciate the nature around you. You might even practice the Sa Ta Na Ma meditation while you are walking to bring yourself into a state of awareness and calm.

★★★

Any reminder you can give yourself to simply *be* will bring you to the place where you sit in the home of your Self. Your heart, nervous system, and entire body will thank you, and so will your whole family as they are able to sense the peacefulness emanating from you—both through looking at you and by feeling your calming presence.

Creating New Neural Pathways

When the intention is to come home to your Self, using tools of mindfulness, yoga, meditation, self-love, or other available resources, you begin the gentle process of releasing the old neural pathways that have outlived their service to you as you evolve.

Do you know that you can create new neural pathways at any time during your life? Scientists used to think that there was a window of time in which neural pathways were created, but now we know that they continue to be formed throughout life. The good news is that you can journey into new internal territory at any stage of life, no matter what habits and patterns are present in your brain right now.

Neural pathway development is explained by Dr. Gene Van Tassell, contributor for the educational website Brains.org. He says, "The more often a pathway is used, the more sensitive the pathway becomes, and the more developed that pathway becomes in the individual brain. As these pathways develop, the collective group of used pathways become a map of how an individual thinks, reasons, and remembers. Neurons which are not stimulated in these pathways tend to wither away and become unusable. These neuron cells either die or change in ways that render them ineffective."[10]

Similar to walking a path through a forest, the neural paths in the brain that are worn are easier to travel. But if they don't take you to a place where you really want to go, then you have the choice to make an effort, little by little or all at once, to turn in a different direction—one that barely resembles a path to begin with. With a focused mind and intention in the heart, you begin the work, labored at first, then easier as time goes on. You courageously begin the expansive work of creating new neural pathways that bring you into alignment with who you truly are.

If you develop a habit of moving into these new neural pathways when things are going well, it will be easier when life seems to be pulling you in different directions. You may find it helpful to think about how the new neural pathways strengthen each time you use them. Take it a step further and visualize the old paths drying up and the new ones getting easier to find!

Moving Out of the Old and Into the New: A Practice

With a focus on creating new neural pathways, these yoga exercises and postures are designed to activate the body's spinal fluid as well as the more subtle energy, called *ojas*. Once activated, this vital energy circulates through all your organs, wakes up your brain, and helps you move into new, positive directions.

---

10. Dr. Gene Van Tassell, "Neural Pathway Development," www.brains.org/path.htm.

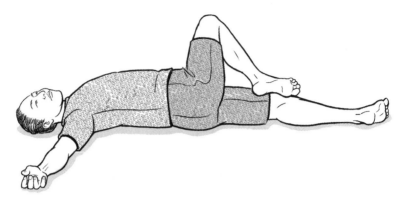

Figure 5a: Cat Stretch

Cat Stretch: You know how flexible cats are, almost like they have no bones in their bodies? Well, this is their secret—the Cat Stretch! Lie on your back on either the floor or a firm bed. Draw one bent knee up toward your chest. Exhale as you bring the bent knee across to the other side of your body, and gently lower the knee toward the floor in a lying spinal twist. For a deeper twist, bring your arms out to the sides of your body on the floor and turn your head to the opposite side from your bent leg (figure 5a). Hold the position and breathe for a minute. Then switch and repeat with the other leg.

The benefits of this movement are that it releases tension in the lower back, pelvis, and legs.

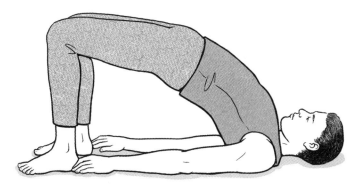

Figure 5b: Bridge Pose

Bridge Pose: Still on your back, bend your knees with your feet flat on the floor. Tuck your pelvis forward slightly to release pressure from your lower spine. Your arms are resting by your sides. Inhale slowly through your nose. At the same time, engage your abdominal muscles as you begin to lift your lower spine off the floor. Then smoothly continue inhaling as you lift the spine, vertebra by vertebra, from the floor. Lift as high as you can without strain. Your neck stays on the floor or bed (figure 5b). At the top of the inhalation, pause the breath for a moment. Then exhale slowly through your nose as you begin to lower first the upper spine, then the middle spine, then lower. Progressively curl the spine back to the floor, ending in the starting position. Repeat several times.

This exercise brings flexibility to the spine, allowing energy and spinal fluid to move freely through the spine to the brain and all parts of the body. It also tones and strengthens the abdominal muscles and the back.

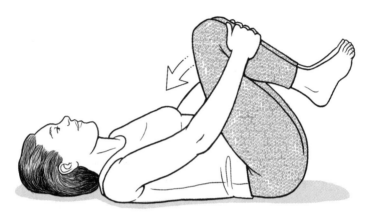

Figure 5c: Knee Tuck

Knee Tuck: While lying on your back, bring both knees up toward your chest. Wrap your arms around your shins while pressing your knees toward your chest (figure 5c). Take a few deep breaths in and out.

By doing this exercise, you will experience a good counter-stretch, which allows the back and hips to relax after arching in Bridge Pose.

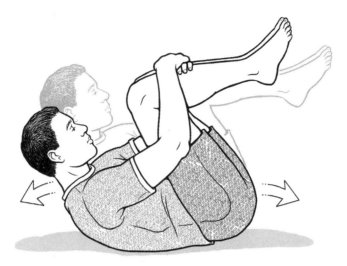

Figure 5d: Rock

Rock: With arms around the shins and knees to chest, rock up and down on the spine a few times and sit up (figure 5d).

Aside from being a natural way to bring the body from a prone position to a seated position, this exercise also enlivens the spinal fluid.

Meditation: Stress Relief
and Clearing Emotions from the Past

Sit in Easy Pose with a straight spine, or as an alternative, you can sit on a straight-backed chair with the spine straight. Place the hands at the center of the chest, with the tips of the thumb and each of the fingers of the left hand touching the tips of the thumb and each of the fingers of the right hand. The hands will form a type of tent or teepee. There is space between the two palms, and the fingertips are pointing upward (figure 5c).

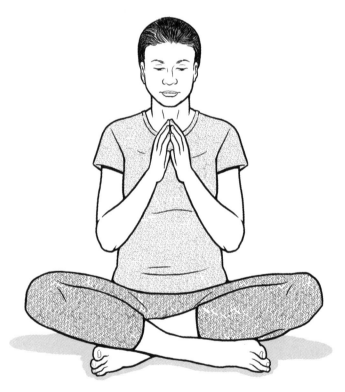

Figure 5e: Meditation

The eyes are mostly closed during this meditation, but you'll want to look softly toward the tip of the nose and beyond. Breathe four times per minute: inhale for five seconds, hold for five seconds, and exhale for five seconds. Practice for five to eleven minutes or until you feel relief from stress.

This meditation is especially useful for dealing with stressful relationships and with past family issues. It addresses phobias, fears, and neuroses. It can help to remove unsettling thoughts from the past that surface in the present and then release them into the hands of the universe for resolution.

Children's Practice: Butterfly-Cocoon

While lying on your back, draw your knees into the chest as you breathe out. This is the Cocoon Pose (figure 5fa). Then breathe in and extend the legs straight out from the body, with the toes pointed, at an angle that is about two-thirds of the way from the ground. At the same time, your arms extend straight out to the sides but not touching the floor. The palms are open. This is Butterfly Pose (figure 5fb). Continue the movement; exhale into the Cocoon position and inhale into the Butterfly position.

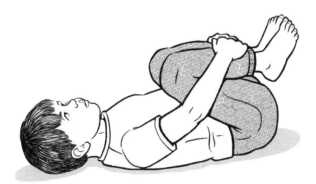

Figure 5fa: Cocoon Pose

Parents and teachers are invited to do this exercise along with the children. Children of all ages may practice this, although very young children may not have the abdominal strength to hold their legs out for more than a few seconds, which is fine. Since this is a back-and-forth motion, no position is held for more than two to five seconds.

This exercise is really beneficial for helping to organize and strengthen the nervous system, making it particularly useful for those who get nervous or anxious or who startle easily.

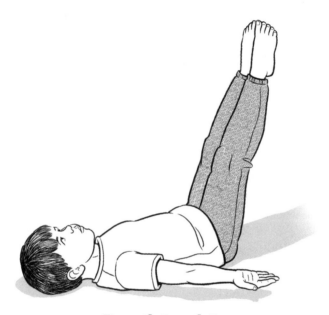

Figure 5fb: Butterfly Pose

When you are doing Butterfly-Cocoon, it can be a helpful repatterning exercise for the Moro reflex (where a startled look comes over the face and the arms and legs extend out, much as if the infant were falling), which is a reflex that is normally integrated as an infant. However, there are times when this reflex does require further integration through childhood and even adulthood, and Butterfly-Cocoon can be a good remedy.

Chapter Highlights

- **If you have been gone, it's time to return home:** Remember that as we age and the world persuades us to act and behave in certain ways, the way we are meant to be—our authentic Self—is always with us, and in this place, we find home.

- **Your greatest friend is you:** The one relationship that is pivotal in bringing success to your other relationships is the one that you have with *you*. Through finding acceptance and peace within yourself, you can prepare yourself to be a parent, friend, and partner to others in a more meaningful way.

- **Find ways to stay connected with your child-self:** The child in you is rooted in your authentic Self. Find and refamiliarize yourself with the child within you, as this will help you to see things from a fresh and honest perspective—one that is free of the opinions of others and society in general.

- **Just say no to the momentum machine:** Stop in a moment of awareness and ask yourself, "What is the cost of all this fast-paced living? Is it worth it?" Most likely, if you are in the home of your Self, or at least in the vicinity, the answer will be to slow down, reevaluate, and find out what is really important in the big picture.

- **Remember that your heart is just as smart as your mind—or smarter:** Scientists have discovered that the intuitions that come from our hearts actually inform our brains, so the more we honor our heart's wisdom, the more we come home to our Self.

- **Always be mindful of the moment:** It is helpful to know that there are times when our reaction in the moment may not be to the moment itself, but to something else that we've let linger. When we lose sight of the moment, we lose an opportunity to connect to and understand the situation from our authentic Self.

- **Strengthen neural pathways for positive experiences:** The more we use neural pathways, the stronger they become. When it comes to creating positive habits of thought that take us into a place of deeper connection, it can be helpful to remember that as we strengthen the new habits, we strengthen the neural pathways, and that eventually the old unhelpful patterns and pathways will become less accessible.

CHAPTER 6

The Wonderful Side of Being Different

One day some years ago, I was at the local community center and struck up a conversation with a father who was there with his family. Like many parents, he had dropped off his child for swimming lessons. As we talked, Greg, the father, shared with me that his ten-year-old son, Nick, had autism. I mentioned that I had a connection with children and yoga and that I offered workshops on "Autism Yoga." With this information, he began to open up about his experiences with autism, seeing that I might be able to grasp some of the daily struggles that children with autism (and their caretakers) have.

Greg shared that when Nick was a baby, he and his wife found out that he had autism. It was so scary for Greg and his wife. He had no idea how hard it would be, and watching Nick develop "differently" was tough. Nick didn't have language for many years, then finally he began talking. However, Nick knew no differently, and Greg found that being with him was always so special because of the interesting way he looked at life. A pivotal moment for Greg was when he made an important realization. He told me, "It's funny, but at some point I realized that if I had a choice about whether he would be like a regular kid, or as he is, that I would definitely choose him as he is." Greg said this last part with the biggest smile coming straight from his heart. Seeing this type of genuine expression really demonstrates just how important the successes in our lives can be, whether they are large or small. For Greg, I'm sure hearing the word "daddy" was a triumph that was just as great as if he'd just climbed Mount Everest.

Greg continued to share his insightful story: "Nick thinks differently and sometimes it blows me away. Like one time when I was really stressed-out and going through some hard times with my work. Nick and his brother were in the car with me. We were getting ready to drive somewhere and they were fussing at each other. I told them I had a short fuse and needed them to calm down. Nick moved up to the front seat without a word, fished through my CDs, found one with no label, and put it on. He said to me, 'Put on track three.' It was Whitney Houston singing 'The Greatest Love of All.' It was just what I needed to hear. I lost it and just cried, filled with such emotion and happiness. How did he know? I don't know. He just is special that way. I guess it is the autism. I don't know."

As Greg shared these intense thoughts with me, I was so appreciative of him entrusting me with this beautiful story. In giving back, I told him something that made him smile, something he could take with him and remember when times got hard with his son. I said, "In our work with children and yoga we have a saying that goes like this: *Special needs? Maybe, but we prefer to think of them as children with special intentions!*"

Children with Special Intentions

All children—and, in fact, all beings—come into life with purpose, so the idea of special intentions is true for all of us. The children we meet or hear about whose brains seem to be wired differently from "typical" children are here to show us a more dramatic demonstration of what many of us feel to a lesser degree. For example, we have mostly learned to adapt to the bombardment of noise and visual stimuli at a social gathering, but a child with sensory sensitivities might scream and run over to a corner to hide, covering their ears to block out the chaos. From the so-called normal point of view, the child's action may seem extreme. But in truth, the action is a direct response to what the child is experiencing on the inside. Furthermore, it would be the response most of us would have if we had not learned to numb ourselves or tune out the stimuli.

Rather than referring to children with sensory differences as having issues or disorders, I choose to use the term "sensory-special" when referring to them. A label or category is necessary at times for clarity, but I believe that our labels can be honoring and empowering. My aim in working with sensory-special children, as it is with all children, is to give them yoga and mindfulness tools to soften oversensitivity and better function in everyday life while continuing to honor their unique abilities. Thinking of them as having *unique abilities* is key because it helps us turn our attention to the positive rather than focusing on perceived *disabilities*.

How do we best assess ourselves when we are interacting with a child who has been diagnosed as sensory-special? I've found that through asking ourselves key questions that pinpoint our intent and action, we have a good chance of truly being present in the situation. Think about:

- How am I viewing a child who has been diagnosed as sensory-special?
- Do I see a label with that child, or am I truly seeing the child?
- How well am I able to be a neutral presence to observe what it is the child experiences?

***

From decades of working with sensory-special children, I can testify that there is a wide range of attributes that are commonly found, and even more when considering all the possible combinations of those traits. In fact, generalizing about children with sensory differences and how they might behave is nearly impossible. It is good to remember that just as we long for others to see us as individuals, so do these exceptional children.

I love being with children with these special outlooks, because I have discovered that they are good examples of how I might live my life in a more authentic way. I appreciate how they seem to have their own agenda and care not at all or very little about what others think. Most of the children I've seen, especially those with autism, are not wired to think about social niceties. Personally, I find this way of being so refreshing; it's like taking a deep breath while standing by the ocean. They help us remember that it is less helpful to care so much about others' opinions and more helpful to care about what brings us happiness and wholeness. Can you see how relying on what others think actually takes us away from our own inner guidance? These kids are good teachers, showing us how to let go of others' opinions so we can hone in on what it is that calls to us most strongly. Because of their ability to do this, these children can be more strongly tuned in to their inner guidance than almost anyone.

Everyone can get fixated at times and create challenges for themselves as well as others. For these children, the challenge may be in trying to get dressed in the morning or lining up for lunch at school, or any number of tasks that are part of daily life. If we can take a breath and realize that a challenge is a learning moment, our intuition begins to flow and solutions come. Maybe the message is to slow down and be a little late for an appointment, while making a mental note to plan better for the next time. Maybe it is to sing a song that catches the child's attention, and during the song, the task at hand gets done. There are as many ways for our intuition to bring us insight and solutions as there are stars in the sky.

I find it exciting that sensory-special children mostly function from an energetic framework. It seems like they are using their intuitive right brain more than their academic left brain, like they truly are differently wired. They respond more to the energy or feeling of the interaction than to the words or actions themselves. All children are much more aware of these higher levels of energetic frequencies than adults are, and this sensitivity seems to be heightened in children on the autism spectrum. I am reminded of something Yogi Bhajan once said, a statement that has resounded with me all throughout this journey with children and yoga: "Children are super-sensitive, full-fledged people, with high-potency antennae, which record every vibration in their vicinity, completely and very deeply." This statement is beautifully accurate in describing the sensory-special children I've had the good fortune to interact with, as well as most of the "typical" children we interact with.

***

Allison, my partner in the training program for children with sensory differences and a long-time occupational therapist, works in several school systems in her county. Upon a teacher's request, Allison was called into a classroom to observe a rather rambunctious three-year-old girl, Nina. Nina was always running all over the place and was unable to focus on one thing for very long. This obviously gave her teacher concerns, and Allison wanted to explore ways to make Nina's classroom experiences more meaningful, and less disruptive—for everyone's sake. Nina's parents were equally eager to figure out how to better connect with her and relay their expectations of her behavior.

When Allison went into the classroom, she observed the class from the back of the room, not interacting with Nina but simply observing her behaviors. She wanted to observe two things:

• How Nina approached play and engaged in it
• Who Nina interacted with and in what ways

Nina did fit the criteria for a child in need of therapy, so it was decided to give her sessions outside the classroom environment where they could work with her one-on-one.

With the one-on-one approach to her therapy, Nina didn't really show any signs of improvement. Everything was continually prompted and she still couldn't sit still. Furthermore, her "regular" classroom environment was not really effective for her. The mentality of the others in the classroom was more like, "When will Nina be at her session so we can have some type of normalcy?"

Allison sensed this concern immediately and saw how it was counterproductive to the results that everyone wanted for Nina. She changed the directive for Nina and went back to the classroom, simply observing her from the distance again. There was no interaction between Nina and her at this time. The goals were still the same: finding a way for Nina to be present in the classroom and be a part of it in a more constructive, focused manner.

Through all the observations, Allison saw endless suggestions she could give, including putting Nina in a smaller group. However, she understood that this idea would not solve the problem, but would only teach Nina how to adapt to that environment. Nina needed to find solutions that came from within her for how to calm herself down and settle into the appropriate behaviors for her classroom. In turn, this would naturally carry over into activities outside of that room.

The best way that Allison could do this was to become a source of really good, grounded energy herself. This meant she had to do the following:

- Drop all clinical thoughts.
- Come up with meaningful goals that were specific to Nina.
- Make sure to focus on Nina in the present, not bringing in any past or present influences from other evaluations or observations about her.

In Radiant Child Yoga, we have a saying that you *are* the yoga that you bring to everything you do. And in her work, Allison has a habit of grounding herself into this space of *being* yoga—united in body, mind, and spirit. As she prepared to work with Nina, she took some time to meditate and breathe deeply before she even entered the classroom. As she did this, Allison felt the energy inside of her change, and it became calmer and more positive. She truly understood that if she wasn't threatening, she'd have a much greater chance of reaching out to Nina in a more effective way. Her thoughts included things such as *Nina, I don't want you to be any different than you are. I'm coming to this interaction with no expectations, just to be with you in this space.*

One factor about the classroom setting that had to change immediately was the one adult who was acting almost like a guard, making sure that Nina physically stayed in her seat. Allison had this adult leave first, knowing that she couldn't create the connection with Nina with that kind of energy influencing the situation.

Allison went and stood behind Nina, and focused herself on a singular thought: *I am just here to observe Nina, to have fun doing what preschool kids do.* Her breathing was calming and her mind quiet. There was no expectation other than to observe.

Nina sat there coloring just like the other kids, not needing any prompting or redirecting from Allison. Nina's behavior was dramatically different, as she usually had to be corralled into her seat by a hovering adult. The other kids didn't take notice of this, but Nina's teacher did, wearing an expression of "what's happening?" on her face.

This technique was so simple compared to some types of observation and therapy that were fundamental to Allison's professional training. It was really just a matter of her being present in a soft and quiet manner, which Allison had learned to embody from a consistent yoga and meditation practice, as well as from her firm foundation in the perspective that we are vibrational beings.

Only after the activity was done did Allison bend down next to Nina, remaining quiet and connected to Nina as a whole being, a soul. Nina looked at Allison from head to toe, taking in her presence. Finally she said, "Wow! You have a very nice shirt!" Those were Nina's first words ever to Allison, and afterward she asked, "Can I go with you?"

The success that Allison saw led the other adults in the room to take note. Some appreciated her work in silent amazement, and others thanked her. Nina's parents were eager to understand how Allison had done this, since they were very receptive to learning the techniques that would help them better guide Nina. It really was a beautiful achievement, because it helped everyone realize that it wasn't that Nina wanted to be a disruptive child; she just didn't understand how to go about being anything else. It was obvious that she was sensitive to the feeling-energy of those around her, and having calm, centered people around who accepted her as she was made all the difference.

Allison's example is wonderful and insightful and, according to her, only one of many examples of things that children have taught her. I understand this feeling deeply and passionately because it's this type of communication and inner awareness that I always am inspired to bring to children, whether through yoga or just by being a calm and support-ive presence, as Allison was with Nina. When you work this way with children, it becomes clear that children determine on their own if they are safe or not, depending on the energy the adults bring to the situation. It is good for all of us to ask ourselves as we interact with children, *Am I geared toward changing this child? Or am I simply and purely being here for this child, with no agenda of my own?* If a child senses that the adult is simply there to change them, a barrier will likely be created in an instant—one that is easy to build and much harder to break down.

★★★

Life is about finding our joy, and we actually do this best with other people. That's why people like Allison set such a good example for all of us, reminding us that our first job with children is often to make them feel comfortable with who they are, as they are. Allison's ability to "be the yoga" in order to create this connection is beautiful and radiant, and is something we can all do as well.

Helpful Guidelines for Parents and Caregivers

Feel free to add to this list of helpful tips that I've compiled based on my work with children on the autism spectrum and those who have been diagnosed with ADD/ADHD. These tips may be helpful for working with all children, since they are based on treating each child as an individual, without concern for categories or diagnoses:

- Get on the level where you can look eye to eye with the child. Have a smile on your face that is genuine, because children can sense our true emotions and gestures. Remember that they are visually oriented and feeling-oriented. Many times they cannot express what they feel, so the most successful interactions happen when the adult is mindful of subtle messaging from the child. If there is discord or disharmony among people, parents, and teachers, for example, children who are sensitive to feeling-energy may begin to act out or suddenly change behavior. Often they do not consciously know what caused the reaction and cannot verbalize their feelings.

- Slow down … way down. In our fast-paced world, we don't even realize how fast we are thinking, moving, and multitasking. And for what? It's a good question to contemplate. It can help you see the craziness that we often think is normal, and you will automatically begin to slow down.

- Communicate only the necessary "now" step. Speak only the most necessary words to get the job done. For example, say to the child, "Shoes on now." Show with your body. I quickly learned about this when I was teaching a yoga class to a group of children with autism, many of whom were nonverbal. I found that I had to slow down and stop talking. When I wanted them to stretch out their legs, I exaggerated the motion and used no words. I thumped my hands on my legs, tapping from the thighs down to ankles to show how to stretch. I pointed to my nose and exaggerated the inhalation, then blew out strongly through my mouth, and gave a big smile. I became a yoga mime—and it worked! They followed my lead within their individual abilities.

• Be predictable. Children need routines to feel safe, and those with sensory integration differences need it even more. In the yoga class I just described, we repeated the leg stretching for approximately two minutes, until I saw the first signs of group restlessness and inattention. In the following week's class, I'd do the exact same routine, and possibly use visual cues, like cards with simple illustrations of each pose or exercise.

• Look for something going well. Look for what is possible for them to do first, and then begin to invite them to take the next step in becoming independent. Always let a loving message shine through your expression and words, and be mindful of holding an energetic space of positivity. Give up measuring them against an academic or behavioral standard. If you'd like to measure, let your standard be how well the children are able to guide themselves into a joyful, internally connected space.

• Train your mind to let go of thinking in terms of diagnoses. As Allison demonstrated, being in a state of yoga means mind, body, and spirit are one whole, and we are grounded in that wholeness. A great way to lead yourself into "being the yoga" is this: when interacting with a child with a diagnosis or with obvious sensory differences, take the child's point of view and imagine the child asking you, "Do you see my diagnosis or do you see me—the being I truly am?"

• See what moves them—what they are interested in. Then use your creativity to introduce an activity that is similar. For example, a child who is rocking or rolling on the floor may enjoy doing a Bundle Roll exercise (see the end of this chapter), or rolling like a log, or rolling up into the yoga mat. On the other hand, if it seems wise not to interfere, allow them to come up with their own activities. Being attuned to what is happening at that moment is important.

- Allow them to set the tone and pace for their routine as much as possible. As the need for new ways to school these children, as well as all children, has arisen, there has been a rise in school systems and methods that focus on natural sensory integration, like Montessori schools, Reggio Emilia schools, and other choices where children guide themselves in learning, while the teachers use logic and intuition to guide the children.

- Allow yourself to go into their world. Find out what is so fascinating about rolling back and forth on the floor, what sensory stimulation is taking place. Go to where you see everything for the first time and discover the magic that happens when the light switch is turned off and on, over and over. Any number of experiences that we might consider mundane can be looked at with new eyes and hearts when we go into the world of the child. As Maria Montessori said, "Follow the child."

- Offer children a heart-centered connection, honor them as they are, and give them the sense that *it's okay, you are fine*. This is one of the most magical ways to receive an invitation to their world. These qualities of love and acceptance are what we all crave in our lives, so these special ones are inadvertently teaching us to work on an energy level instead of a clinical level, because oftentimes the energy level is what will work!

***

As talked about in the story of Allison and Nina earlier in this chapter, the most important thing you are doing when interacting with children is not something you actually do; it is something you *feel*. We are often not aware of what we are actually feeling in the moment, which can become our greatest obstacle. To overcome this, try this experiment.

1. Take a breath and then read these sentences: *Something went wrong. We have to fix it.*

1. Close your eyes and acknowledge how you feel after reading these sentences.

2. Now take another deep breath and then read these sentences: *Everything is okay. It's okay.*

3. Close your eyes and acknowledge how you feel after reading these sentences.

4. Breathe in deeply and calmly again.

Did you notice what feelings rose up within you after reading each of these sections? The first two sentences promote discord or even panic. The second two sentences bring relief and harmony. Which feels better? Which do you want to cultivate in your life in general and specifically with regard to children? Since how we feel is how we vibrate, it makes sense that we would want to feel good for our own wellbeing and also because we want the signal or energetic message we are sending to children to be positive.

★★★

Find the Fascination

Once when I had traveled out of town to give a children's yoga training, I was visited in my hotel room by a concerned mother of a nonverbal three-year-old boy who appeared likely to be on the autism spectrum. She wanted me to show her how she could help her son in general and specifically with yoga. As soon as the boy entered the room, he made a beeline for the air conditioner mounted on the wall. He didn't acknowledge the presence of either his mom or me, but was totally fascinated with the mechanics of the machine.

In reaching out to draw him into the yoga, his mother and I invited him to join us in a few poses and songs, but he didn't seem interested. Our efforts were going nowhere because he had his own agenda, as many little ones do whether they are sensory-special or not. He proceeded to spend a full fifteen minutes in the kitchenette, rolling the silverware drawer back and forth. I knelt down by him so I was at eye level with him, curious to see what he was seeing. He paid no attention to me, repetitively opening and closing the drawer. For a few minutes I allowed my adult mind to go, so I could be present to what he was finding so interesting. I was not just trying to be present; I *was* present. Just like this little boy, I saw the wheel turning in the groove inside the cabinet as if for the first time, and for a few seconds I was enchanted. At that exact moment, he turned to look at me directly in the eyes and smiled, confirming that, yes, we were on the same wavelength. That was the highlight of the experience for me. The hard part was helping the distraught mother find connection and joy with the behavior of her son. I understand that these things can be frustrating; we all get frustrated at times. Not all challenges are welcomed, but there are always gifts in challenges, whether it is growth or awareness or just "being."

I never saw or heard from that mother again, but it is my great hope that our meeting helped to plant a seed within her so she sees her son as "okay." As this small boy goes into his world, may she go with him, discovering a delightful connection that she never knew existed.

Grounding Gifted Children

Sensory-special comes in many different forms. Children who are considered to be gifted or exceptional are often hypersensitive and need some special considerations. Ram Das was one of these little ones. He had such a strong sense of empowerment and dignity even at a very young age, and for the most part, he was not slow to express his true feelings. One such story is about how he hated being called "cute." Between ages one and two, I would wheel him around the neighborhood in his baby carriage. Sitting up straight, holding onto the carriage bar, and looking around at everything, he looked so bright and beautiful that people were attracted to him and wanted to meet him. Sometimes the only thing they could think to say was how cute he was. When he heard that, he would scowl at them, and they'd be taken aback. I would then have to deal with my own conflicting feelings—the social pressure

I felt that Ram Das should "make nice" with people versus wanting to honor his response, which I believed was based on his non-acceptance of being objectified. It was a tough decision, but one that I couldn't just solve by telling him what to do. However, I still wasn't sure how to handle it exactly.

By the age of two, he was articulate enough to confirm what I had suspected. After one of these incidents, I squatted down in front of the stroller and, in a very open and connected way, asked him, "Ram Das, what is going on?" He said, "I don't like 'cute.'" Okay, I understood that. I asked, "What would you rather they say to you?" This was an answer that was truly of interest to me, so that I could have a clearer understanding of the way he perceived life. His answer astonished me. Ram Das said, "They can say I'm handsome." I didn't even know that he knew this word, but his self-dignity resonated with the concept, while "cuteness" did not resonate.

Understanding Our Needs

Like many parents, Kate has always been involved and eager to help her son, Aidan, seek out environments that help him become the happiest and best that he can be. Aidan was a very creative and excitable little boy, prone to bursting in on Kate and sharing whatever thoughts were on his mind at that given moment. This habit proved to be disruptive at times, motivating Kate to develop a great way to help Aiden become more aware of how he approached others with his infectious enthusiasm. Kate came up with a concept that she called "your thought bubble, my thought bubble."

With this concept, if Aidan came into a room eager to share, Kate would say to him, "You're in my thought bubble right now. In a little bit, you can come in, but not right now." This was a concept that the highly intelligent and imaginative Aidan could really relate to. It also became quite clear that Aidan had more going on. He was also hypersensitive and hyperactive, as well as bright and talented.

By second grade, things became more emotionally traumatic for Aidan. Because of his intelligence, Aidan was moved up a grade, but his social and emotional development was below his intelligence level. The result was that he became disruptive and began acting out in class. Desperate, Kate had some neuropsychological testing done on Aidan. The result was that Aidan was determined to have a sensitive nervous system. The testing helped them to understand the situation better; however, solutions were not easy to come by for a family living in a large metropolitan city, with all its overstimulation of the senses.

The doctors recommended activities such as rock climbing, aerial movement, and other activities that would apply pressure to the joints or to the entire body. By chance, Kate and Aidan happened to go to a Cirque du Soleil show around that time. Aidan was absolutely drawn to it, and a week later, he was practicing some of the same moves that he saw the performers doing in the show. This was their solution!

They found a circus school for Aidan, and he loved everything from the aerial feats to climbing and using his naturally highly flexible body to accomplish the goals. Eventually, he was accepted into a performing youth troupe, which also served to give him a sense of belonging to a community. The most exciting benefit that Kate found, however, came from a more emotional place. She saw Aidan go from sad to happy, because he now had a channel for his boundless energy and creativity.

The circus school didn't solve everything for Aidan, though. He still had problems with school. After a lot of research, Kate found a school with a different philosophy: *We encourage students and teachers alike to think outside the box and find ways to view each student as an individual.* This ideology allowed Aidan to finally find the connection that helped fulfill his intellectual and emotional needs. It was a huge step forward, allowing him to move at his own pace and not just try to fit into a mold that was not made for him.

As all the pieces started to fall into place, Kate quickly found out that structure and predictability formed a stable foundation for Aidan. This included bedtimes, mealtimes, and even when and where Aidan did his homework. Every morning Kate would wake him up with the same words and run down the list of what Aidan needed to know for that day. When inconsistency occurred, it filled up Aidan's brain with too much to process. With structure, he could focus on what was going on inside his body and how he was feeling.

One thing that became apparent to Kate was how her own internal state was directly linked to the wellbeing of her son. If Kate had a bad day, Aidan was likely to have a bad day as well. The way Kate handled this was to remember a phrase: *keep it simple.* This helped her to avoid internalizing all the things that she couldn't control. She became more aware of her energy—how her thoughts were portrayed and how her words were interpreted. Even something as simple as talking about taking a shower could change the tone of a day if not done in a thoughtful way. This is how Kate became highly aware of the power of her thoughts and words in ways that most people wouldn't imagine to be necessary or even possible.

Today, Kate describes parenting as a spiritual practice, and I believe that's a wonderful way to view it. She's had to dig deep into her well and give up certain things she never thought she'd have to, including a high-profile career. However, in the end, Kate's determination to be the best parent she could be drew her back into her own self to address certain things she'd experienced and felt. Over time, she was able to heal much of her own history and find an inner strength she never knew she had. Without Aidan's "problems," this likely never would have happened. It was the gift that Kate's special gift, Aidan, gave her.

Diverse Souls within One Universe

Many times we spend so much time dwelling on *why* a child is a certain way that we forget what an amazing being the child actually *is*. In appreciating a child, we open the door to understanding what resonates with that child, and we are better able to help the child maximize their potential, as Kate did with Aidan.

As you reflect on your own child or the children who impact you in some way, whether personally or in your professional life, take some time to better understand their vantage point. Here are some things to keep in mind:

- Children are very aware of the vibrational energy that comes from the adults around them.

- Sensory-special children respond to their environment in ways that are consistent with how they perceive the world. As adults, we can help them realize that they are just the way they should be, amazing in their own way. Different is not bad, and we find the gifts in "different" when we honor the differences.

- Striving for conformity can lead to challenges if we do not approach children as individuals. Rarely does a strictly clinical approach address the individuality of a child, and even more rarely does it acknowledge the inner being—the heart and soul—of the child.

- Through children, we are given incredible opportunities to understand ourselves better, and through their challenges, not only can we help them in a meaningful, deeply connected way, but we can also help ourselves. Our tools are yoga, meditation, mindfulness, and an overarching intention to live, as much as possible, in our own authenticity, for our own sake and for the sake of our children, who learn best by example.

Every being has a radiance in them that has the potential to shine so brightly that we are drawn to them as if they were the sun in our universe. In children, we can experience this in its original, authentic form and walk away with a deep, unspoken understanding of their—and our own—magnificence.

Raising Your Energy Flow: A Practice

From Kundalini Yoga comes a practice known as Sat Kriya. A *kriya* in yoga is a complete action, and *Sat* means "truth" or "authenticity." You will chant the sounds of *Sat* (True) *Nam* (Beingness). Feel that you are declaring the truth of who you are with every repetition of the mantra.

This practice elevates you into your true Self through the circulation of internal energy through all of the body's energy centers, called *chakras*. It also brings balance to your mind, body, and spirit.

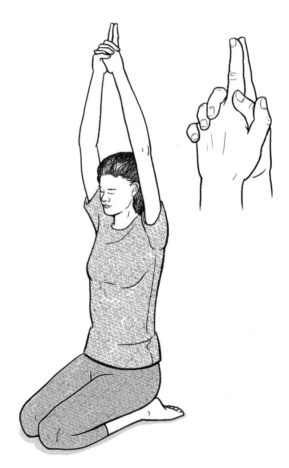

Figure 6a: Sat Kriya

1. Sit on your heels if possible. If not, sit cross-legged or with your spine straight in a chair.

2. Interlock all the fingers except the index fingers of each hand, which are pressed together and pointing straight up. Stretch the arms up straight overhead, with the elbows hugging the sides of the head. Maintain an upward feeling and lengthening of the spine the entire time (figure 6a).

3. Close the eyes and gently bring your focus to the forehead, where the nose and eyebrows meet.

4. Exhale strongly with the sound *Sat* (rhymes with "what") as you quickly pull the navel up and in toward the spine. This movement is similar to the way the belly presses sharply inward as you are blowing your nose, for example. The sound should be very powerful but not necessarily loud.

5. This next part is all one movement. As you relax the belly, allow for a quick, short inhalation (through the mouth is fine) and then say *Nam* (rhymes with "mom"). "Nam" is short; the syllable is not extended. It may be barely audible.

6. Chant emphatically in a constant rhythm about eight times per ten seconds for a few minutes.

7. To end, inhale and suspend the breath inside the body. Squeeze the muscles from the buttocks all the way up the back, past the shoulders. Mentally allow the energy to flow upward and through the top of the skull. Hold for five to ten seconds, then exhale and relax.

8. Ideally you should relax in Child's Pose (figure 6b) for at least the same amount of time as you practiced Sat Kriya. If this is not comfortable, lie on your back instead (figure 6c).

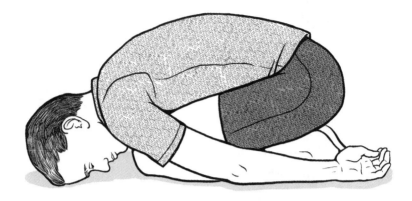

Figure 6b: Child's Pose

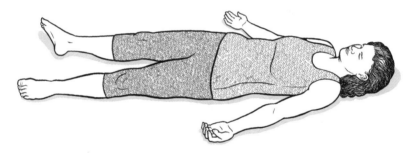

Figure 6c: Relaxation on back

Besides raising the energy flow of the chakras, so you feel more up-lifted and ready for life's challenges, Sat Kriya improves your general health, since all the internal organs receive a gentle, rhythmic massage from this exercise. Because Sat Kriya is a powerful yoga technique, beginners should practice it for two to three minutes. After a period of steady practice, Sat Kriya can be extended incrementally over time up to a maximum of thirty minutes. Since this is a powerful practice meant for adult bodies, children under the age of eleven should not practice Sat Kriya. I suggest that youth ages eleven to thirteen practice it for one to two minutes per session. Youth ages fourteen to eighteen may start with two minutes and work up to five minutes.

Bundle Roll Children's Practice

Demonstrate this exercise before having children practice it. Lie down face up on the floor on a soft surface, either on a dense carpet or on several yoga mats placed next to each other lengthwise. Stiffen your body and raise your head and upper body as well as your legs about six to twelve inches from the floor. Point your toes. Begin to rock side to side until you gain enough momentum to roll over (figure 6d). Take advantage of the momentum to continue the rolling as long as you would like, then reverse and roll back to where you started.

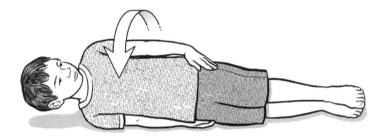

Figure 6d: Bundle Roll

Here are a few tips on performing a Bundle Roll. The secret is in gaining momentum before you roll and keeping the body tensed the entire time. The head will naturally stay out of the way as you roll; the head and face will not touch the floor. You may find it natural to exhale as the body's front side contacts the floor.

The intensive tightening of the body helps to strengthen and organize the nervous system and creates an effect that is similar to swaddling. Wrapping a person from the shoulders down to the legs using stretchy "body socks" is a technique that has been used effectively in what is referred to as "deep pressure therapy" for sensory integration. Additionally, as the body contacts the floor while rolling over, an instant release of tension naturally occurs, similar to what happens during a full body massage. This is good for proprioception, which is being able to feel where one's body is in space. The Bundle Roll is great for adults as well as children.

Log Roll: A Yoga Story

This is the Bundle Roll with a story line! The children gather at one end of the room, and while waiting for their turn to roll, the children stay focused by imagining that they are trees along the shore of a river. They stand in Tree Pose, with one leg bent and placed on the other leg. Younger children may want to stand in Low Branch Tree, with the bent leg close to the ankle (figure 6e).

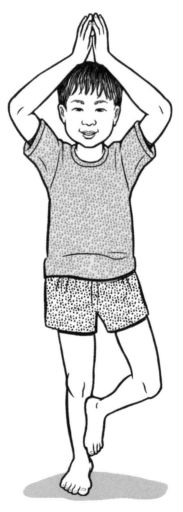

Figure 6e: Low Branch Tree

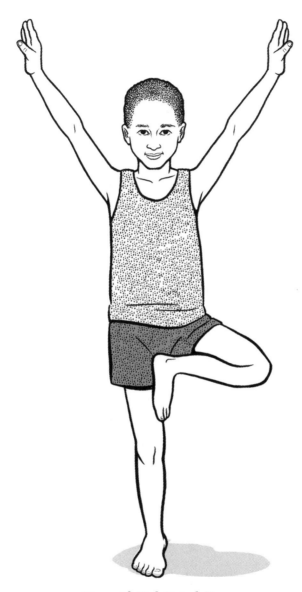

Figure 6f: High Branch Tree

Older children may want to challenge themselves with "high branch tree," in which the bent leg is pressed against the straight leg above the knee (figure 6f). The arms are up, with the palms together or apart.

One at a time, the children become logs by doing Bundle Roll and rolling across the "river," which is the length of the room. Once on the other side of the river, they become trees once again, this time standing on the opposite leg.

Chapter Highlights

- **Embrace how our uniqueness gives us value:** In relation to children with "special intentions," we can best work with our fears when we honor the uniqueness that we find within our own being and in children. It is through this acknowledgment that we find the innate joy in every individual we choose to connect with.

- **Be careful not to label people:** Labels are necessary sometimes, just to give us a perspective or frame of reference. However, children with sensory needs often display a wide range of characteristics, so one label does not fit them all. In fact, we are all that way.

- **The more we complicate communication, the tougher it can become to be understood:** There are times when simple, direct language is necessary. Not every interaction needs an elaborate explanation for it to be understood and processed. Don't lose the heart of your message by filling it with unnecessary details.

- **Stability creates the grounding that children need:** There is comfort in routine and knowing what the expectations are, regardless of who you are. When we remember this, we can create a nurturing environment where everyone understands their role and embraces their contributions within their family and for the betterment of their own lives.

- **Relinquish your desire to focus on "why":** There isn't always an instant explanation for everything, but there is always a way to accept what is. From there, you find the wisdom to "just be," without placing stressful expectations or emotions on situations. Often the solution flows in unexpected ways once we come to a neutral, grounded center of acceptance.

CHAPTER 7

Giving Children Space to Grow

In the spiritual community I lived in for many years, Yogi Bhajan often commented on parental attachment. One of his sayings was particularly impactful for me, and to this day, it is one that I pass on to my students. He'd say, "The little tree cannot grow in the shade of the big tree." He often spoke about how children need to have space to question, to investigate, to experience, and to learn for themselves. His teachings about the stages of children's lives included acknowledging the following:

- In the first three years of life, children are deeply influenced by maternal energy.
- During the second three years of life, they are more influenced by paternal energy.
- By the age of seven, children are people in their own right.

Through observation and experiences within my own family, the concepts of Yogi Bhajan have played out, much in the manner in which he described them.

By the age of nine or ten, many children in our spiritual community have gone to school in India for nine months of the year, Ram Das included. As a parent, it was very hard for me to have him away during the school year, yet I was comforted by knowing that the India experience would serve him the rest of his life, considering all the incredible life skills he was learning.

Our living situation, though unusual, still brought about many of the same experiences that a regular home life might. All children, despite their age and proximity to their parents, can have their own experiences and interactions apart from their parents. For example, going to preschool or daycare or spending the weekend with grandparents serves to give young children space to grow. They get to see how other people think and act. They begin to understand that there is a big world out there, one with a huge variety of lifestyles and attitudes, and they naturally gravitate toward finding their place in this world.

There is much we as parents and teachers can do to encourage independent thinking and self-reliance at all ages. Even taking a question that a young child asks and thoughtfully discussing it together, hearing their viewpoint before giving our own, can be a way of honoring the wisdom that young people so naturally express. The subtle message we impart is this: *You are capable. You are your own person.* Along with sending that supportive message, nothing is more valuable than leading children to discover their own guidance. Easy access to our inner guidance is what we all are looking for, and these little ones are wonderful examples for us since they are so naturally connected to their inner wisdom.

Many of the parents and teachers I work with have a trusting attitude toward the inner wisdom of children, like the parent of one of my five-year-old students, who wisely took advice from her daughter. The little girl would calmly say, "Take a deep breath, Mama!" whenever she found that her mom was getting upset. As we've said before, these kids are big souls in little bodies!

Emotions in Flow

Strong emotions rise up when we think about those we love, because we so deeply want to keep them safe from harm, both physically and emotionally. In yogic teachings, emotions are often described as *energy in mo-*

tion. Have you noticed how emotions naturally flow one into the other in response to thoughts and ideas? This emotional flow could be thought of as your vibrational stance, or the energetic position you are taking at any moment. Try to be aware of this as much as possible, as it will help you find guidance in any given moment.

Imagine that you are at home preparing a meal in your kitchen when suddenly an ambulance siren goes off close by your house. The intensity of the sound can trigger a strong, startled reaction within you. That is a natural initial response, and after the initial startle reflex, you have several choices: (1) stay in hyper-alert mode, with shallow breathing and an elevated pulse; (2) be curious and possibly check out the situation from your window; or (3) go back to homeostasis by taking a few deep breaths and continuing with your work. Your response depends on what you believe about the situation. Basically, it is your vibrational stance. Do you view the siren as something to be alarmed about? Do you feel curious or alarmed? Do you allow yourself to calm down after the initial startle reflex so you can go back to that peaceful place and continue your food prep?

The last choice—of noticing, allowing, and moving into what you prefer—is the yoga way of working with emotions. When in a quiet frame of mind, you may notice the interplay of mind and emotion. Emotion flows in the form of sensation in your body/mind. If you play with the flow of sensation in meditative ways—for example, by using the guided meditation practice near the end of chapter 2—you will discover that it is possible to allow sensation to morph, unimpeded by any resistance you may habitually offer. Conversely, you may also allow the sensation to be as it naturally is, without energizing it with your thoughts. Allowing is the first step in becoming a conscious human being. It means not influencing the situation, but just feeling what is there. You can tell yourself, "I am where I am on this issue, and that is okay because I know it will evolve if I let it *be*, let it speak to me, and give myself space and time to find the gift in it."

Children learn what they live, as well as what they witness the adults around them living. In my Montessori training, we called this phenomenon the "absorbent mind," especially with reference to children between zero and six years old. Small, seemingly insignificant incidents, like the way the adult responds to the siren, are actually important because, consciously or unconsciously, children draw conclusions about life from the beliefs and attitudes of those around them in everyday life.

In order to get a feel for the transformative power of making internal shifts, I invite you to experiment with *allowing*. Begin with something easy, such as a small comment that someone makes about you that just doesn't sit right, or a chronic behavior that you wish your child did not have. Don't energize the feeling by gathering other similar thoughts from your past or by steeling yourself against the feeling. The monster in the closet just gets bigger when we push it away in fear. When we relax with "what is," we create space around the issue—and not only does this space bring us peace in the moment, but it also makes room for creative solutions to flow into our awareness.

Staying Steady Through Emotional Times

Izabela is a long-time yoga teacher who specializes in working with children and is also a trainer for my program. While Izabela has found tremendous value in teaching yoga poses and exercises, she knows that there is a vital element required for teaching children that is above and beyond the yoga practice. She keeps close to her heart this teaching from the Radiant Child Yoga manual: *to hold an intention of the highest wellbeing on every level: body, mind, and spirit for the children in your care and yourself.*

According to Izabela, "When children are anxious and fearful, this intention has empowered me to become a non-anxious presence, not only in the children's lives but also in my own."

Remaining steady is not always easy to do, but we can draw inspiration from how Izabela handled an incident that happened while she was teaching a children's yoga class in a private school. There were about ten children in Izabela's care, ages four and up. They were about to start, sitting in a semicircle, when all of the sudden there was a lot of commotion outside of the classroom. Doorbells were ringing over and over, and raised, nervous adult voices could be heard. It was a distraction that could not be ignored. Jeremy, Izabela's co-teacher, went into the hall to investigate. Izabela heard someone say, "Car accident! Call the ambulance!"

Although the children in class were young, they were aware of the sense of panic in the adults' voices and understood those words enough to know that something bad had happened. They huddled near Izabela, anxiety and fear showing on their faces. Then, to make matters worse, another teacher entered the room with about twenty more children and announced, "Everybody has to stay with Izabela. Don't leave the room." Then she left, leaving Izabela with about thirty children, none of them older than ten. She sensed their anxiety and nervousness increase, and some of the children looked ready to cry.

In the intensity of the moment, Izabela's feelings of anxiety also rose. Thankfully, she became immediately aware of her feelings and remembered that children are super-sensitive to the emotions of adults. She knew she had to project a calm and reassuring presence in an authentic manner to help them through what they were experiencing. She gave a warm smile and opened her arms, inviting the new children to join the yoga circle. "It is wonderful for you to be part of our yoga class today," she said in a cheerful and calm voice.

The children gladly sat down, and Izabela said, "Please sit with your legs crossed, and then take hold of your outside ankle. Pretend this is your saddle. We are going to ride our bumpy camel across the desert. Breathe in deeply as you stretch forward...Now breathe out...Keep moving and breathing. Now go a little faster. Remember, it is very hot in the desert, and we want to get across it quickly!"

She saw smiles flashing around the room and felt the energy change from being anxious to relaxed. Then she finished the warm-up routine with the song "Fly Like a Butterfly," which is part of the Radiant Child

Yoga program. The children embraced this song with excitement, and it became a wonderful way to help their minds travel to a beautiful place, one in which they were laughing with each other as they talked about what kind of butterfly they would like to be and places they would like to fly to. Next, Izabela enthusiastically said, "Let's go on a little adventure."

"Yes!" they shouted. Then they were off, jogging through the jungle, pretending to be all kinds of animals, traveling through the tall grass, and walking like crabs.

Typically at the end of the animal adventure, everyone lies down in the relaxation pose; however, with the situation right outside the room, Izabela's guidance told her this would not be effective at the moment. Instead, she decided to continue with a wonderful Radiant Child meditation called "I am happy" (which will be discussed in detail at the end of this chapter). Upon hearing this song, every child gave Izabela their complete attention, imitating her movements and repeating the mantra after her: *I am happy, I am good. I am happy, I am good. I am, I am, I am free! Happy, happy, happy to be me!* The children's enthusiasm gave Izabela confidence that everything was going to be all right—everyone just had to believe in themselves—and that message was able to be relayed effectively to the children because it rang true for them. In quite a natural and nurturing manner, the children showed how truly amazing they were and began to help lift each other up as they sang. When their teacher reentered the room, the environment was noticeably different. The children were chanting *I am happy, I am good. I am happy, I am good.* This wonderful new energy was created within about a thirty-minute time period.

Despite the very stressful situation, Izabela had stayed with her intention of bringing a deeper sense of peace and calm to everybody in the room, even those not familiar with yoga. According to Izabela, "Every time I am given the joy of being in front of children to share yoga with them, I strive wholeheartedly to convey positive and encouraging subtle messages through my thoughts and feelings. That is conveyed in the use of cheering words, engaging and fun activity, and my own emotions and body language. The children's response to the positive energy is truly magical!"

Being a Non-Anxious Presence

Not all of us have Izabela's wonderful insight to remain calm in anxious situations. Also, it is often easier to stay calm and centered with other people's children than with our own. Many of us do what the little tree analogy suggests: we give more sunshine space to those who are not so close to us and more shade to those who grow next to us. None of this is intentional, of course; it's just that sometimes our attachment gets in the way. Our emotional heart gets very attached to those we love, and that is most apparent in the relationships we have with our children. Whether they are born from our wombs or from another womb, they are ours ... or so we think. I like to remember the parenting wisdom offered by nineteenth-century poet Kahlil Gibran: "Your children are not your children. They are sons and daughters of Life's longing for itself. They come through you but not from you, and though they are with you yet they belong not to you."[11]

Even within the same family, each child has their own dreams, challenges, gifts, and personality. Each comes here not to complete the parents' dreams, but to complete their own destiny. Even as I am writing these words, I know how entangled I am with my own son. While I love and wish the best for the two children I raised, each for three years, they do not elicit the same emotions that my relationship with my son brings forth. It seems to me that the combination of knowing him so intimately from birth and observing the characteristics he has that intertwine with my own (for better or worse) has created a deep attachment as well as a deep love. One thing I am discovering is that the better I clean up old, unhelpful beliefs and patterns within me, the better the relationship between us becomes. Simply put, without all that excess baggage, there is more space within me, and thus there is more space between

---

11. Kahlil Gibran, *The Prophet* (New York: Alfred A. Knopf, 1923), p. 17.

us. And on the good days, the space gets filled up with loving, apprecia-tive energy instead of emotional attachment. However, we don't always have "good" days. Knowing what to do on a rougher day is important, too. For me, it is a matter of embracing the opportunity to reflect on what was off balance and what belief system I was operating from that was out of alignment with my authentic Self. Thus begins the inner work of neutral noticing, gaining insight, and moving in the direction of making different choices next time.

Our emotional hearts are so intertwined with our children's lives. It is natural to love and want to protect our children, but there is a distinct difference between protecting and overprotecting them. Most parents interfere with their children's lives more than is healthy for either of them. Why do we do this? I see us as wanting to be helpful—we want to save our children from pain and danger. So how can we protect and guide our children and still be a non-anxious presence for them? We need to do the following things:

- Find our own non-anxious place inside ourselves.
- Realize that children need space to investigate and to learn and know things directly for themselves.
- Learn to find a balance between the negative mind and the positive mind, and come to experience the neutral mind.

All of the tools given in this book will help you become a calmer, balanced person with an expanded perspective on children as "big souls in young bodies." Here is a simple suggestion that may help you get a real sense of what I'm talking about. At a time when you are feeling relaxed, happy, and connected to your authentic Self, get on the same level as the child you are interacting with. Look into the child's eyes, and allow a genuine smile to come to your eyes. From this energy frequen-cy, speak to the Big Soul in front of you, no matter what form it comes in. Even if the child is crying, angry, or indifferent, accept it all. Feel you are actively holding that moment in a loving embrace.

You may like to first internalize and then project the feeling of this message: *I accept all of you, and I am in vibrational alignment with the best of you.* In this frame of mind and heart, it is likely that you will have a noteworthy, if subtle, experience with the child. And more importantly, you will learn something new that changes how you view your relationship with children: you will gain the ability to be in a space of loving non-attachment, honoring the soul in front of you as a being connected to you yet separate from you. From that experience, trusting the natural inner guidance and wisdom of the child comes easily.

Because of their simplicity and natural instincts, animals can be great teachers about balance. Animal parents are vigilant providers for their newborns. Yet as their young become ready for and interested in independence, animal parents naturally take a backseat, holding a stable and non-interfering role until they are satisfied that their young are ready for the world.

Yes, we can all benefit from taking parenting cues from the natural world. Sometimes, though, a parent will discover that their own vulnerability has impacted their desire to be a natural parent. Such was the case with Lindsey.

Parenting from the Heart, Not the Hurts

When Lindsey's daughter Tara was born, Lindsey decided that she and her husband, Brad, were going to do everything possible to create a nurturing environment for her. They would take emotional cues from Tara to decide how to handle every situation. Tara would always be carried next to her mom or dad. Lindsey would limit how much time she was apart from Tara, so that they were together as much as 98 percent of the time.

By the time Tara was a year and a half old, it began to dawn on Lindsey that her life revolved completely around Tara. Lindsey slowly began to realize that she was so desperate for Tara to feel loved and appreciated that she was almost a slave to Tara. She felt she had given herself up, as though she didn't exist as a person but only as Tara's mother. In Lindsey's words, "I never gave myself permission to say no to Tara. I thought it was horrible if she cried, so I did dances so she wouldn't cry. I tried to keep her happy at all costs. I sacrificed my own wellbeing, the wellbeing of our family, and even my relationship with my husband."

Partway through the second year of Tara's life, Lindsey got very ill, and so did Tara. They went to a naturopathic doctor who was recommended by a friend. The doctor told her straight out that she was "reactive parenting," meaning that she was reacting to her own childhood hurts by parenting her daughter in an unconscious attempt to rectify her own past. Lindsey was shocked. More than shocked—she was horrified. Her thoughts were, *I am a nurturing parent! How can I be a reactive parent?*

But then she realized that the doctor had spoken the truth. Lindsey had been viewing her daughter's life through the eyes of her own hurt inner child whom she was still carrying inside. She was determined that Tara's life would be different, but she had taken it to an extreme because she had not healed her own inner child. It was hard for Lindsey to face this, but somehow she drew up her courage and realized it was exactly what she needed to hear. The doctor pointed her in the direction of inner work to heal herself. Lindsey found some excellent support in a wonderful counselor whom she saw for nearly four years and who guided her on her path to her soul. As Lindsey faced her inner sadness and anger, Lindsey and Tara both healed and regained balance in their relationship.

To help her cope and flourish, Lindsey adopted many of the tools that are in this book: yoga, meditation, mindfulness, journaling, energy work, and, most especially, a spiritual counselor whom she could consult regularly. All of these processes have helped her to befriend herself more lovingly and allow old beliefs and patterns to fall away. In her determination to be who she really is—not the hurt child, but the totality of her authentic Self—she now feels more connected and balanced than she ever thought possible. Lindsey expressed this beautifully when she shared: "So now I ask myself, am I still off balance? Are there still more ways I can be living and parenting from my heart and not from the hurts? I have come so far! I have opened up my heart and let go of the hurt that kept me so deeply locked in protection mode. As a result, Tara became less attached to me in that highly emotional way. She responded to all the inner changes I made with so much grace and ease. It freed her to be more her true self, so she was no longer reacting to all the fear, anger, and sadness I had been living in. It has changed our everyday life. For example, in the past, when Tara spilled her juice, I would feel rage rising up in my body and she would feel it too. Now it's much more subtle, and I may make a joke about how well she spilled something. When I do that, any last traces of rage diffuse, whereas before it exploded out of me energetically before I even had a chance to choose differently. That's really it: I get to choose much more now and it is so refreshing. I feel myself respond to life from a more compassionate, graceful place, instead of from anger and inner hurt. I feel so blessed."

Lindsey's courageous story is inspiring to all of us who have blind spots, and who among us does not? We all want the best for our children, but sometimes we are unconsciously living our lives through our children. During the eight years that Ram Das went to school in India, I was learning to be a non-anxious presence for him. I found that many beliefs held in my emotional heart had no foundation once I listened to the voice of my authentic, broad-view Self, who had this to say:

- If you subscribe to the idea that the world is a very dangerous place, you will thwart your child's ability to experience life directly and come to his own conclusions.
- If you subscribe to the idea that your child is vulnerable, you cannot see his strengths and intuitive capacity.
- If you assert your beliefs and opinions to your child when he is not asking for your input, you superimpose your guidance on his own

inner knowing, and he will come to either replace his innate guidance with yours or resent you for not supporting his own guidance.

• If you cling to your child in pride, he will struggle to be free because
he innately knows that he belongs only to his Self.

★★★

Since we want to be in balance, we must acknowledge that the negative
or cautionary mind plays an essential role. I am not saying that parents
should throw caution to the wind. What I am referring to is balancing
the negative mind and the positive mind, and in turn, balancing both
with the neutral mind. The neutral mind is the witness to it all. It understands the pluses and minuses of each situation. From the stable place
of the broad view, the neutral mind will give you an accurate read every
time.

Attention Without Apprehension

Kartar has always amazed me with his ability to come to the neutral
mind. Here, in his own words, he tells how his emotional attachment to
our son could have caused him to slide into fearfulness. Instead he sur-
rendered to his authentic Self and held a space for Ram Das to experience his own indomitable spirit. In Kartar's words:

> In June of 1995, our family arrived for a yoga gathering in the dry
> heat of the high New Mexican desert. The three of us decided
> to go to Bandelier National Monument, a scenic state park built
> around the cliff dwellings of the ancestral Anasazi Indians. To re-
> ally see the caves, you have to climb twenty, sometimes forty, feet
> up rough ladders made of hewn logs with rungs that are tied on
> with leather wrappings.
>
> Even at the age of four, Ram Das was an eager explorer and
> climber. We went up the ladders with Shakta going first and him
> going second. I was right behind him so that if he fell back, I
> had him covered. The trouble was that he was so small that he

could fall right through the openings between rungs. I shook the thought away and paid keen attention, feeling determined to remember that it was his adventure and not mine to spoil.

When we got to the top, Ram Das fully explored the caves, even going out to the edges where the drops were thirty to forty feet. After a series of these climbs, we followed some paths through the valley and arrived at a place where there were a number of dwellings high in the cliff. These were probably a hundred fifty feet or more from the ground, reached by a series of these same kinds of ladders staggered up the cliff.

As soon as he saw these dwellings, Ram Das said, "I'm going there!" His determined response thrilled me, but at the same time I was thinking, *Oh my God, this is for real!* We started up the first ladder, with Ram Das climbing without hesitation up every one of the ladders, moving quickly from climb to climb. I was behind him the whole way. We fully explored the caves and then climbed back down, rung by rung. We did it all and it became a day to remember. It was the day when Ram Das's love of climbing and exploring came bursting forth without the least bit of fear. The details are vivid in my mind to this day, and I'm forever grateful that I could be just in step myself, letting go of the fear, taking the high road, and trusting his inner guidance and my own!

Letting Children Learn from Life

Understanding that children have their own soul wisdom also allows us to step back and see that they have their own soul lessons, or karma. Our own meditative minds can give us the inner discipline we need so we don't interfere with life lessons that children are learning. I often see parents and teachers, myself included, seeking control, but in reality the control we are seeking is the control of bringing our own selves back to center, into alignment with our authentic Self. I've noticed that once I get even a glimmer of that alignment, I drop the agenda that I was pressing, whether it was with my child, my husband, or one of my coworkers. Some helpful reminders that have worked for me over the years are these words of wisdom that I picked up from masterful teachers and my own masterful inner teacher:

- There is only one relationship to attend to—the one between my self and my Self. All other relationships are secondary and depend on the primary relationship to my Self.

- My perception of reality makes up my experience of reality. Making "feeling better" the prize I am reaching for changes how I feel. Then, through the Law of Attraction, changing how I feel changes what I experience.

- What am I giving airtime to? Am I giving airtime to the problem or the solution? Am I thinking and talking about what I *don't* want or what I *do* want?

It is very enlightening to realize that the solution and the problem are two different vibrations, and you can't get to a solution by being immersed in a problem. They are like two different channels on your TV set. When you turn your attention to the vision and feeling of what you want, and really feel it, you will have deactivated the vibration of the problem. Remember, worrying is praying for what you don't want. I've always loved the truth and humor in that statement!

The Stories We Tell Ourselves

I have found great benefit over the years in the work of Abraham-Hicks. In their many books and videos, Esther and Jerry Hicks talk about getting ready for the relationship you want to have with your child (and others) by practicing the feeling of it until it becomes your predominant vibration. When you look for things in your real life that "match" the energy of where you want to go, you will increase the feeling within you and the signal you are broadcasting will attract to you what is a match to that. These words are empowering and give us, their recipients, strong and positive emotions.

We can begin to tell a different story about the relationship we have with a child, whether the child is our own or not. Take time to meditate on the story, and during that time, listen closely to what your inner knowing tells you instead of focusing on the circumstances of the story. Pay attention to the feeling, and lean in the direction that feels better. At the moment you choose to feel the happier place, even if it is just a bit happier, you are on your way to a better story.

In *Ask and It Is Given* by Esther and Jerry Hicks, there is a written process called the Focus Wheel that has become a great tool for me and for many of my students and friends.[12] To begin working with the Focus Wheel, you think of something that you want to feel better about than you currently do. You turn your attention to what you know you *do* want as a result of clearly knowing what you *don't* want. This better-feeling space—or vision—is what you write in the central circle of the Focus Wheel. If you have difficulty figuring out what goes in the central circle, ask yourself, "I know what I *don't* want, so what is it that I *do* want?" Think of this statement as a feeling place that you'd like to move into. This central statement cannot be something that you want someone else to do, because you cannot vibrate for another being, meaning you cannot make someone else do anything. However, you have absolute ability to choose your own vibration, and you do this by feeling what it is you actually want to experience—and this becomes your central statement in the Focus Wheel.

Starting above the central circle, and moving in a clockwise direction, you write statements that you believe are true for you, ones that feel true and good in relation to your central vision. Each statement is a spoke in the wheel, so the diagram looks like a central sun (your vision) with rays of affirming statements supporting your vision. The intention is that, as you move around the wheel, you continue to feel better and

12. Esther and Jerry Hicks, *Ask and It Is Given* (Carlsbad, CA: Hay House, 2004), p. 247.

closer to the feeling of the statement that you've placed in the center circle.

You don't write down goals or plans of action. It will not work to write something you wish for but don't believe; in that case, you will be faking it, and you will know it is not true on a feeling level. When you know you are on the mark with this process, whatever you write down will either bring you a feeling of relief or will feel good to you as you think about it and write it.

I recall creating a Focus Wheel at a time when I was feeling discord in my relationship with a sixteen-year-old Ram Das. There was agitation between us, some of it because of household duties not getting done—a pretty common theme between parents and children! So I knew what I *didn't* want; that was easy. And what *did* I want? Was it just to get chores done? Yes, in part, but it was more than that. I wanted us to have a more positive, harmonious working relationship. Realizing this helped guide me to what I wanted to write. In the central circle I wrote these words: *Lightness and harmony with my son.*

I wrote the following succession of personal truths after closing my eyes and taking a few deep breaths before writing each statement. Because the "spokes" around the wheel begin at the top and move clockwise in a natural progression, I could feel the positive momentum charging my statements. Each statement led to the next, and they all seemed to wind around with an upward-moving momentum. By the time I got to the last one, I marveled at how, once again, this insightful process and my own inner guidance had led me to a wholly satisfying conclusion:

Vision circle: *Lightness and harmony with my son*

1. *I am getting better at noticing when I am ready to "pounce."*
2. *When household and other duties are not done, I am getting better at noticing my reaction before speaking or taking action.*

3. *I don't exactly know the solution to this situation, but I feel I am getting closer to knowing. I am on the right track.*

4. *I know if I keep on the track of appreciating our time together—no matter how brief—that the other parts will change, too.*

5. *I can feel that both of us want a lightness and appreciation with each other, and we both know how to get there because we've done it many times.*

6. *When I am feeling good with him, I am not sweating the small stuff.*

7. *In the times when we are all having fun, there is a lightness. There have been many times that he did his duties without me saying anything, even with enthusiasm.*

8. *I am looking forward to discovering more lightness in the relationship with my son.*

The process took about a half-hour. I clearly felt myself moving into a different place by the time I got to the last statement. I knew I could handle myself in a flowing, authentic way, and the resulting interaction with my son was exactly as stated in the vision statement: more harmony and lightness, which resulted in a natural flow in getting household duties done.

Almost always, the harmony we seek and the outcomes we desire can manifest, even if we are feeling frustrated. It is a matter of us directing our path in a loving and nurturing way to ourselves, which is then conveyed to others through our energy and presence and not just our words or even actions.

Natural Discipline

Speaking of engaging cooperation with children, there are really excellent skills to be learned from Faber and Mazlish's book *How to Talk So Kids Will Listen & Listen So Kids Will Talk*. The authors offer simple, helpful tools that create cooperation with children. As a mother and someone who works with children, these tools have proven to be quite beneficial. I have also discovered something I call "natural discipline." This is a phenomenon that usually occurs when I am either

1. stepping back and letting life step in to give children the natural consequences of their actions without any input from me, or
2. enjoying children as they naturally are and letting a sense of order and discipline flow from that space of connection.

Allowing children to experience the natural consequences of their actions encourages them to take responsibility for themselves. When we don't go out of our way to interfere with the learning that comes from experiencing natural consequences, we develop a parenting style that is neither authoritarian nor permissive. Instead, it is one that supports loving adult-child relationships where everyone learns to take responsibility for their actions. Here's a typical scenario that most parents can relate to:

Your child forgets her lunch box for the third time in as many weeks. The first two times, you went out of your way to drive the lunch box to school in time for her lunch hour. After the first two times, you let your child know that it would not be possible for you to take time from your workday in the future. So this third time, you make yourself unavailable, and you let the natural consequences kick in. Your child will not be hurt by this experience—just a little hungry. With the uncomfortable result of that forgetting, most likely your child will take responsibility for her lunch box from that time on.

It is often easy to enjoy children as they are, particularly since they have an innate ability to find fun wherever they go. They naturally make things interesting, despite how they may seem to us from our adult perspective. Have you seen a child just playing with a stick in the dirt or making a car or train out of a discarded box? They are experts at playing with life, and along with that, a natural sense of order and discipline unfolds. How does this come to fruition? In children, I see expertise in the ability to respond properly to the vibrations around them. We can have great relationships with them if we ourselves are more playful while simultaneously creating soul-to-soul connections.

Here's an example. For some years, I was a guest teacher for after-school yoga classes in several schools in my district. Being a guest teacher, I made the rounds to each school, where as many as seventy elementary school children would be introduced to yoga for the first time. In the largest of these one-time classes, the children had finished the energetic, playful style yoga that I teach. They were lying down on the carpeted floor of the gymnasium for deep relaxation.

At the end of this time, I typically use a soft puppet to wake each child, after giving them instructions that when they feel the puppet's touch, they can stretch quietly and sit up without disturbing their friends. For me, these moments are wonderful, because it is often the only opportunity I get to spend time with each child individually. In the few seconds that I interact with each child, I honor the beauty of each one, and add my own loving energy to theirs. As the puppet touches them on the shoulder, I whisper with a smile and a song in my voice, "Wake up now!"

In this particular class of seventy children, it took me about ten minutes to complete the circuit. There was absolutely no sound in the room during those ten minutes. From what I could see and feel, a peaceful space had been created as the children experienced the honoring that passed between us as I moved around the room. They held the space quietly and respectfully until everyone had the chance to feel it.

Off to the side, the teachers and after-school counselors sat and observed, with jaws dropped and amazement on their faces. Was this the same group of rowdy children they often encountered? Yes, it was. After the class was over, a couple of the teachers came up to me, still looking dazed, and said the obvious. "How did you do that?" I thought about it for a moment and said, "You know, I didn't really do anything except create some magic. When you create something magical with children, they want to be part of it. Magic has its own natural discipline."

The Lighthearted Approach

Through all my experiences, I have found that the ideal sort of "discipline" is the type that doesn't feel like discipline. It is approached from a lighthearted space that is deeply rooted in spirit. This type of harmonious space doesn't happen all the time, and that makes it even more precious when it does. Here are some guidelines that I've found helpful for creating a magical, lighthearted space with different ages of children:

- **Simple fantasy play:** With children who are imaginative, generally ages three to nine, make bedtime or naptime more fun by creating a fantasy world under the covers. Get into bed and make a "tent" together by holding up the covers with your arms or propping up some pillows. You can even play a pillow game where you put your head on your child's chest while they become a "living pillow," making your head move by breathing deeply. Then switch roles. Making it fun and fanciful will make it magical—no outside discipline needed!

- **Cooperation:** Establish the idea that when we cooperate, we all can have fun and be powerful, too! Think of our five fingers. If each one just wants to do what it wants to do, then we cannot use our hand to hold a glass, or play with a toy, or call someone on the phone. The concept of cooperation can be that *we all work together to make something good, something fun, happen.* One time during a yoga class for children ages seven to ten, they started getting excited and were making so much noise that I found myself shouting. That had to change! I asked them to stop a moment and we reviewed the concept of cooperation. "It has to be good for everyone, right?" I asked in a quiet voice and with a smile. "Yes," the children answered. "Well, right now it is not fun for me because my throat is hurting from shouting." This did get the children's attention and they grew quieter. I could sense they were realizing that it had to be fun for me as their teacher as well as for them.

Because we had established a respectful relationship, the rest of the class went by without me needing to raise my voice at all.

• **Peaceful place:** Reframe a "time-out" spot to a "time-in" place—a peaceful place. Add a beanbag chair to a corner along with headphones and happy, calming music. Physical movement and breathing will create an attitude adjustment. An easy way to do this is to add yoga cards, like the Yoga Warrior Cards from Radiant Child. Allow children to go there when finding peace is necessary. By introducing this idea at a time when things are calm, it helps convey this message: *We all need a space to go to for peace. It is not a problem or a punishment. I trust that your inner guidance will lead you here when you need it, and I may ask you to go there if I feel you need it.* This kind of friendly and neutral attitude will allow children to find their own self-regulation. It might be helpful if they see that you go there when you need to find your peace, too.

• **Give them space:** Preteens and teens can have a peaceful place, too. Usually it is their bedroom. Allow them space, and be respectful of entering it. Breathe deep and be as kind as you can, remembering that they are going through great mental and hormonal changes. For about forty minutes each day, my young adult son will play incredibly loud music in his downstairs mini-apartment. I know that is how he works out, both physically and mentally. If I start to get annoyed because I am trying to work, I will suddenly remember that this is his way of working through day-to-day pressures. Realizing this is a real attitude-changer for me, and I feel thankful that his inner guidance is working so well. Also, I feel thankful that I can take my laptop to the top level of the house and continue working!

• **Sensitive youth:** Making magic with teens and preteens is quite different from doing so with young ones. A few ways of holding an honoring space for teens and preteens include giving your full attention when they feel like confiding rather than asking a bunch of questions, finding time to laugh together, and generally thinking of them as "sensitive adults."

When we don't approach children from an "urgent" place all the time, we prevent defenses from being raised before we even talk. Most often we all can gauge a person's mood just by the way they enter a room—and then if it seems negative, we will often brace ourselves, which is not the energy frequency that will create a good interaction. Being calm and more lighthearted can allow us to deliver messages and find resolutions without first having to break down our own and the other person's defensive barriers. Keeping this in mind saves frustration and creates sounder relationships—and delivers better results in the moment.

Switchback Breath: A Practice

This is an excellent series for you to practice anytime, and it is recommended to practice before the Journaling in Relation to Children (the next practice) process, since it brings a peaceful focus. Feel free to use the Switchback Breath—one that helps you switch back to who you really are—anytime you want to shift from practicing old habits to creating brand-new life-affirming habits.

I highly recommend this practice for young people beginning at about age nine. I have seen how it can be especially centering for teens and young adults, allowing the hormones to balance and the mind to calm. Children younger than nine can practice this; however, it might be challenging due to the amount of concentration it takes to catch on to the breathing pattern.

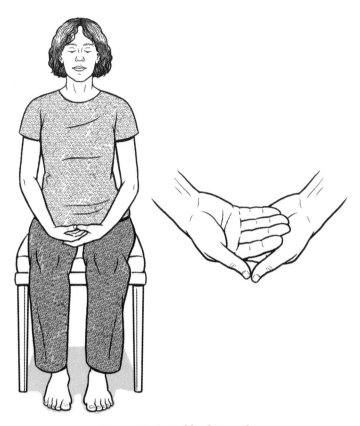

Figure 7a: Switchback Breath

Here is how the Switchback Breath is done. Sit with a straight spine in a chair or on the floor, with your hands resting in your lap, palms facing up. Make a "cup" with your hands by placing the back of your right hand inside your left palm (figure 7a). When you look down at your hands, the palm of your right hand faces you, and the back of your right hand rests inside the left palm in a comfortable way. The tips of the thumbs naturally touch as you sit with your hands in your lap. Close your eyes.

1. Inhale deeply and slowly through your nose, filling your lungs from the base (belly) to the top (upper chest). Pause a moment at the top of the inhalation.

2. Then open your mouth and exhale slowly and deeply. Listen to the sound. At the end of the exhalation, pause slightly.

3. Then inhale through your mouth. At the top of the inhalation there is the slight pause, then exhale through your nose. You are now back to the beginning of the series. Repeat step one and continue through the steps. This is the pattern:

   Inhale ... nose

   Exhale ... mouth

   Inhale ... mouth

   Exhale ... nose

Continue for a period of three to eleven minutes. Then inhale deeply and hold the breath without tightening the throat or face. Sit quietly and let the life force energy, or prana, circulate in your body and mind. Then exhale and relax. Stretch your body to finish.

Journaling in Relation to Children: A Practice

It is suggested that you find a quiet time and space to journal as often as you feel the need, both for your personal growth and to enhance your connection to your Self. In addition, you may find it helpful to journal specifically with the intention of uplifting your relationship to children. The following themes and questions will be helpful starting points toward that end. Take time to write honestly from your innermost, authentic Self.

1. **Serving spirit:** Why do you really want to be with children? How does it serve your spirit? How do you envision your life with children serving their spirit?

2. **Dream on paper:** Create a story/scenario in which you are being with children in the way that you would like to. Feel the feelings, see the scenes, and write about how you and the children respond to each other.

3. **Transforming challenges:** Allow fears, obstacles, and hurts to come to the surface in relationship to being with children. Include whichever of the following are relevant for you: parenting or working with children, transitioning into new careers with children, being with challenging children, or anything that comes up that could be blocking you from living your dream in relation to children. Allow each of the challenges to just be there, and watch them. Then write about them from the place of watching. Use your breath to help you remain in a space of allowing all that comes forward as you write.

4. **Gaining insight:** By allowing and watching our thoughts and feelings, new insights evolve. Write about any insights that have evolved for you today.

5. **Blessing yourself and children:** Affirm your own special gifts and how those gifts benefit children. You may choose to reaffirm them daily, out loud or silently.

I Am Happy Meditation: Children's Practice

As Izabela mentioned earlier in this chapter, children between three and ten really enjoy chanting and making movements to rhythmic chanting, and they love doing this with the "I am happy" meditation. The "chant" in this meditation is in English. In the simplest version of this meditation, the child sits cross-legged and taps out the beat on their legs while chanting the words. For a more comprehensive movement, from the Radiant Child *Yoga in Motion* DVD, the child moves their arms in the following way:

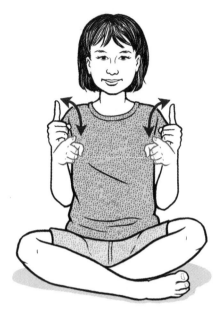

Figure 7b: "I am happy, I am good."

I am happy: Arms are up, with elbows bent and index fingers pointing up. Shake the arms, wrists, and fingers three times, once for the word "I," once for "am," and once for "happy" (figure 7b). This move looks like you are "shaking a finger" at someone.

I am good: Do the same movements as for the previous line.

Repeat the first two lines again.

I am, I am, I am free: Palms are pressed flat together at the belly for the first "I am" (figure 7c). For the second "I am," hands move up to the center of the chest—the heart center (figure 7d).

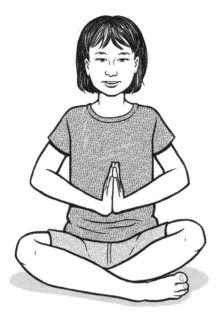

Figure 7c: "I am" (first)

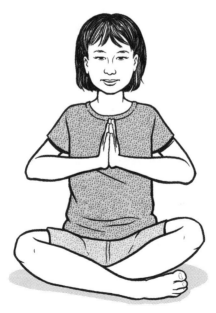

Figure 7d: "I am" (second)

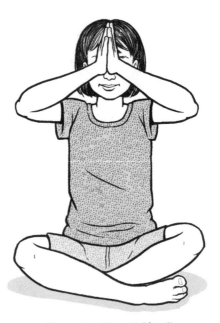

Figure 7e: "I am" (third)

And for the third "I am," the hands move up to the forehead—the
intuition center (figure 7e).

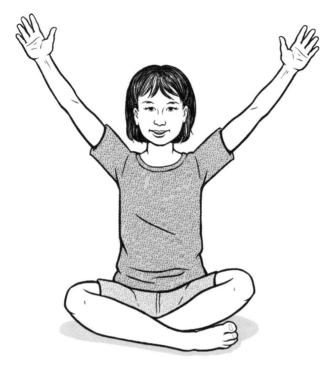

Figure 7f: "Free!"

Then, for the word "free," the arms extend straight upward in a "Y" shape, with hands open and fingers spread (figure 7f).

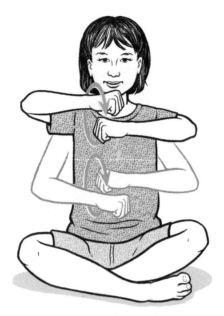

Figure 7g: "Happy, happy, happy to be"

Happy, happy, happy to be me: Starting with the arms overhead, bend the elbows and begin rolling the hands around each other (like the "Wheels on the Bus" song) in a downward movement until they come to the belly for "happy, happy, happy to be," and then on "me," the arms open up, with palms facing outward and fingers spread (figure 7h).

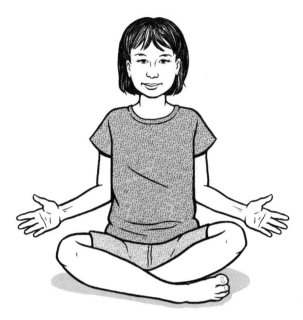

Figure 7h: "Me!"

Repeat this as many times as you like. This practice has proven to be great for bringing everyone, adults and children, back to their happy places!

Note: This is a meditation that Yogi Bhajan gave in the 1980s at one of the children's yoga camps I worked at. He gathered all the children together and told them he was going to teach them a meditation "to teach their parents." He said, "When your parents are not feeling very well or are not behaving well, teach them this little meditation." All of the children loved the idea of being the teacher for their parents, and they have also always loved this meditation for themselves. Out of all the songs and meditations in the Radiant Child Yoga training, the graduates of the program consistently report that "I am happy" gets the most requests from the children.

Chapter Highlights

- **Children have their own guidance:** Let children experiment so they can find their own inner guidance, and as often as possible, come from your own inner guidance when interacting with them. The subtle message we want to convey to children through our words and deeds is: *You are capable. You are your own person, with your own inner guidance.*

- **Children have absorbent minds:** Children absorb attitudes and beliefs in a mostly unconscious way from those closest to them. Developing your meditative mind, being fully present and fully neutral with "what is," and then moving into what you prefer provides an example and a foundation for children's lives.

- **Working with our deep attachment:** We all want the best for our children, but sometimes we are unconsciously living out our lives through theirs. Think of finding a non-anxious place inside you through breath, meditation, or whatever works in the moment. It can be helpful to contemplate the idea that our children come through us to explore their own path and their own karma.

- **The control is within you:** We think we are seeking control of the children in our lives, but in reality the control we seek is that which will bring our own selves back to center and into alignment with the authentic Self. Once we understand this, we can drop our agenda of what we think "has to" happen, and instead feel our way into new ways of working cooperatively with children.

- **Turn in the direction of what you want:** The problem and the solution are on two different frequencies, like two different TV channels. When you turn your attention to the vision and feeling of what you want, you will deactivate the vibration of the problem.

- **Use natural discipline:** This is best done by non-doing. When we step back and allow life to step in, children experience the natural consequences of their actions without any input from an adult. Creating magical connections with children leads to a natural sense of order and discipline.

CHAPTER 8

Be the Lighthouse for Our Children, Our World

We've come this far together, learning how to be present to ourselves, how to move into better-feeling places, and how to connect with our children in meaningful, authentic ways. Now it is time to take the party outside, as the saying goes, by becoming a shining beacon, a lighthouse, for our children—the future of our world. Although it was many years ago, the pivotal question that Yogi Bhajan asked me is still as vivid in my mind as if it happened just last week: "Why do you want to have a child?" When this powerful question led me to an understanding that there really was no good reason, that it would be steered into existence by universal powers or not, I innately understood that my position was to hold a space, a vibration, of readiness without attachment. *Holding a space of light creates a neutral space, a prayer field, that empowers our children and our planetary spiritual evolution.*

We have to ask ourselves and give thoughtful contemplation to what holding a space—holding the light—means. I see it as understanding and living in our own power, and within our own authenticity. Through that vibration, an energetic field of light, love, and truth is created that can be accessed by others.

Think of it this way: When you hold someone as the focus of your attention while you are in the center of your loving, authentic Self, you act as a satellite for them. Even if they are not close to their own center, your satellite beams the way forward, and they have the opportunity to come to center.

Let's go a little further with the idea of energy as light. There is a common saying that there is more to life than meets the eye. If you think about it, all of our senses, while wonderful instruments, have limited ranges of operational frequency. Our eyes cannot see biophotons, for example, which, according to peer-reviewed articles on the National Center for Biotechnology Information website, are known as energy released as light. Scientists have found that the human body directly and rhythmically emits light.[13] In addition, scientists are finding that our DNA communicates with and is created from light itself. It's been observed that DNA produces extremely high biophoton emissions.[14]

Chakras and Children

There is merit to the idea that we are made of light, from the vantage point of both Western science and ancient yogic science. Yogic teachings speak about our energy bodies of light and the whirling wheels of light, our chakras, which are the seven major energy centers of the body. When our chakras are in balance, we feel a balanced state of being—a place where we experience the amazement of being uplifted and grounded at the same time. This is something we have all experienced but may not have been aware of at that moment. As someone with years of yoga practice behind me, I've noticed that I can suddenly become aware of a sensation, perhaps a warm feeling in the throat chakra, which is associated with speaking from a place of authenticity.

13. Masaki Kobayashi, Daisuke Kikuchi, and Hitoshi Okamura, "Imaging of Ultraweak Spontaneous Photon Emission from Human Body Displaying Diurnal Rhythm," *PLoS ONE* 4, no. 7 (July 16, 2009): e6256, doi:10.1371/journal.pone.0006256.

14. F. A. Popp, et al., "Biophoton Emission: New Evidence for Coherence and DNA as Source," *Cell Biophysics* 6, no. 1 (March 6, 1984): 33–52, www.ncbi.nlm.nih.gov /pubmed/6204761.

Sometimes I have noticed a feeling of stagnation or blockage in a certain center as well.

The science of the chakras is a complete study in itself, and one that you may be interested in learning more about. For now, though, let's focus on the fascinating world of children's chakra development from babyhood through adulthood, as explained by the renowned scientist and spiritual intuitive Barbara Ann Brennan in her classic book *Hands of Light.*

Through this book I've been able to gain a greater understanding of these invisible centers of energy. Picture this: a newborn baby has a large and bright crown center at the top of the head where the skull is still open. Imagine this cord of light linking the infant to the spirit world from which he just came. The grounding root chakra at the base of the spine is not well established as a newborn, but it will become more so as the infant gradually becomes a "citizen" of the earth. As the child grows and becomes more of an active participant in life, the root chakra and crown chakra, as well as all the other five chakras, come into balance. For the first years of life, the chakras are all fairly open to outside influences; however, by the age of seven this changes. The child now has a protective covering that serves to screen outside influences so that he is more easily able to absorb or deflect any influences coming into the energy field. As the child matures into a teenager, the chakras and hormones are harmonious sometimes and in upheaval at other times. Finally, as the child grows into an adult, the chakras constantly change to reflect psychological and spiritual growth, culminating in a beautiful lilac color in the energy field surrounding the body as the adult expands from personal love to include love for all beings of the earth.

Having a visual image of the energy field or the chakras may be helpful in our intention to hold a space of light for a child. In this way, we don't have to know what is best for the child in an intellectual way, but we can simply feel and trust that whatever is the best for the person will be able to happen in this healing space of light.

Holding a Healing Space for a Child

I really love making energetic connections with children. I find it exhilarating when we meet in the middle of a beautiful unspoken exchange. For example, once I was teaching a group of school children in a gymnasium. I recognized that one boy was most likely on the autism spectrum. He didn't move at all during the class, but sat with his hair covering his face and the hood of his jacket over his head. As I walked around the room during the deep relaxation section of the yoga class, I held an intention of love and light for him as I passed my hand in an arc about two feet above his head. I could actually feel a healing heat come from my hand as it moved around his energy field. The next time I held a class at the school, he was sitting outside in the hall after class, with the same posture and same hood, but with his hair slightly moved away from his face so that one eye was looking directly at me. I greeted him and smiled, beaming loving energy toward him as I felt myself go into a soul-to-soul meeting with this being. As I turned to go, I said "lots of love to you" and really meant it. He slowly closed his visible eye and opened it again. I took it as a message of acceptance of the connection.

This holding of a space of light, or intention, or prayer, for another is one of the most powerful forms of communication, and is so much more satisfying than a regular everyday conversation. Sometimes we do it out of joy, and sometimes out of necessity. With my friend and student Amanda, her love for her daughter was the catalyst for learning how to hold a space of light for another being.

Amanda's oldest daughter, Sara, was focused on specific interests and was highly sensitive. It was no surprise when Sara decided that she wanted to drop all of her extracurricular activities to pursue what she loved most—dance. She began to devote so much time to it and really shined. Then things started to change.

By the age of thirteen, Sara had become more sensitive to everything around her. Friendships started to crumble. Anxiety started to set in. And even the one thing that had always brought her happiness—

dance—started to present some challenges. Sara would often resist wanting to go to dance class, crying and seeming so afraid, but then Amanda would get her to go and she'd come out happy and transformed. Then the process would start all over again, without Amanda really understanding exactly why.

Desperate for solutions, Amanda reached out to a therapist for help. Amanda was excited to see improvement in Sara after most therapy sessions; however, Sara still said she hated school and felt really isolated when she was there, almost like she didn't belong. That broke Amanda's heart, but what choice did she have other than to be content with the progress, even if it was slow?

Nothing shocked Amanda more than when Sara said that she'd like to go to a boarding school for the performing arts that was sixteen hours away. This was a new concept for Amanda, and one that she'd never considered before. It was contrary to the hands-on parenting she had loved, but she felt she owed it to Sara to let her try. A school where she was with people who shared her passions might be just what was necessary to help her transition into the young lady Amanda saw so clearly when she looked at her. So Sara auditioned and was accepted with a full scholarship. Amanda was proud—and overwhelmed with worry about Sara's emotional wellbeing since she would be so far away. Would she have problems? Amanda found it easier to trust that Sara would be fine, because she also trusted her daughter's instincts.

For the next year and a half, Amanda saw an amazingly well-adjusted Sara, but then, due to some challenges that were difficult for Sara, the cycle started again, but this time the symptoms were different. Suddenly she was calling Amanda a few times a day, compared to once or twice a week. Not only was her emotional health unstable, but her physical health was too, as it was confirmed that she had anorexia.

Everything in Sara's world was becoming more precarious by the day. Somehow, through it all, the light found a way to break through for Amanda and she realized something fundamental: *if she couldn't make sure she herself was good, how could she possibly be strong enough to help her daughter meet these challenges?*

From there, Amanda began to make changes. She began praying and returned to the meditation practices that she'd let lapse since becoming a mother. Knowing that everyone needs support at times, she also began trusting her own instincts about who she could reach out to for helpful nuggets of wisdom. She felt confident that this approach was working, but then it was put to the test in a most unexpected way: the school called and said that Sara's weight had dropped below what was acceptable and that they felt she should be hospitalized. In her heart of hearts, Amanda knew that her daughter hadn't been lying to her about eating what she needed to maintain her weight. She asked the school to reweigh Sara, which they did at a random, unexpected time. And guess what? Her weight was what it had been. The school couldn't explain it—but Amanda could.

There was this warm and loving feeling surrounding Amanda, almost like a warm blanket to comfort her on a chilly day. It was with her while she was at work, and it always lovingly held her, and Sara, too, letting them both know that everything would be okay. Amanda was "telepathically" told that all was well and that she and Sara were safe. *This voice was her inner knowing.*

This meaningful experience helped Amanda grow more committed to thinking positively and not allowing those negative what-ifs to seep into her mind. Her purpose became to share this mindset with Sara, too. Every morning she sent Sara affirmation e-mails. If Sara couldn't sleep, Amanda helped her with relaxation techniques over the phone. She had a specific intuitive way of working with energy by meditating on three qualities: peace, love, and hope. For example, Amanda would reflect on peace until she felt every cell in her body becoming peaceful. She often envisioned peaceful shades of color, such as blue, and she would feel the calming color fill her whole body as she breathed. When she felt that she had fully come into total peace within herself, she would breathe in, gather up the peace in a swirl, and, with an exhalation, envision sending it out of her and into Sara's body and consciousness until she perceived that it had reached Sara and entered into her. She would continue this way, with each emotion having its own unique feeling based on colors and subtle messaging.

After Amanda did this, both in person and from afar, there was always a shift, and while Amanda wasn't certain how she did it, she just knew she had. Understanding how it happened didn't mean as much as the results. *What mattered was that she came to know firsthand that love truly is the opposite of fear, hope the opposite of despair, and peace the opposite of anxiety.*

The first moment when Amanda could not deny that Sara had really come into a better place was during one of Sara's last performances before graduation. She did a modern dance piece, an art form that allows for more creativity and emotional expression, and Amanda witnessed her dance with such emotion and abandon that she was completely captivated in such a meaningful way. As Amanda watched her, so many emotions surged through her and were clearly flowing through Sara's body. Sara came off the stage when she was done and burst into tears. She had given it everything she had, and it was uniquely her moment.

Things seldom heal overnight, and Sara's challenges continued, though to a much lesser degree. Amanda really couldn't say if she had played any real role in Sara's healing, but she sensed how her ability to look beyond what was right in front of her had helped Sara hold steady until her time for healing arrived. Sara received Amanda's unconditional love and she knew that she was trusted, which was huge. Really, Amanda just made certain that Sara knew she believed in her and that she could get well. This was the way that Amanda was a lighthouse for Sara.

As Amanda has learned, and I know that we all can learn, love does heal, and in times of desperation there is always the ability to go inside and pull from the reservoir of our true Self, which then gives us the power to hold a space of light for another person.

Don't Bite the Bait!

As Amanda learned, and as we've all been learning throughout our journey toward an extraordinary life with children, before we can be a beacon for another, we must have our light shining from within. In addition, children provide a squeaky clean mirror for reflecting what we are learning. When Ram Das was younger, we had a saying in our family: "Don't bite the bait!" I used this line countless times as a reminder to him when his temper flared or when he felt victimized by something that had happened. Of course, I needed the reminder just as much as he did. I began to recognize that the "bait" was anything that seemed to throw me off-center. Sometimes I could catch myself before I was "hooked," but not always. If a situation had its way with me, I was greeted by a gleeful, highly enthusiastic Ram Das, who jumped at the opportunity to tell me, "Mama, you're biting the bait. Don't do it!" It didn't take him long to figure out that this was the best countermove for those times when I was reacting negatively to his behavior!

Biting the bait instead of leaving it dangling is a choice we make when strong challenges come up. We have about a microsecond to decide if we are going to react or respond. When we react, we are under the spell of the situation at hand. Our reaction most likely will empower the discord. When we respond, we empower ourselves to stay centered. We take a moment to breathe consciously. We then have a better chance of positively influencing the situation.

Recognize You in the Other

It's a sobering moment when you realize that no one "makes" you feel a certain way. If someone is expressing negativity toward you, no matter how it looks on the outside, you do have a choice. You can react and feel hurt. You can retaliate with your own hurtful words. Alternatively, you can choose to *see the unseen*—that which is not apparent on the surface but truly is the bigger picture. When we choose to see the unseen, we are recognizing our own Self in the other person's Self. We all have fragmented, insecure parts within us, and we all have the potential to live from our innate goodness, our authentic Self. Once you see through the eyes of compassionate understanding, you see that this truth applies equally to you and to the other person. This is what we mean when we say "namaste" as a greeting in yoga; we are verbally and energetically saying that "the light in me recognizes the light in you."

In seeing the unseen, you might even think, *how can I uplift the situation?* If you are responding instead of reacting, you might first be quiet and let the angry words echo so that the other person can hear him- or herself and choose a different response. Or, after acknowledging the strong emotion that was expressed, see if the two of you can come to a solution. The important thing is that you are communicating from your Self to the other person's Self, just like a beam of light illuminates the way through a dark forest and a lighthouse guides ships to safety with its beacon.

What if you don't see the unseen? What if you fall into a hurt or defensive emotional response? This is something that happens to all of us at times. When this happens, you can be your own best friend and accept your reaction as part of a learning curve. You can take it one step further and realize that you had a part in attracting whatever came to you. You can be open to finding out what vibration you were holding that attracted the situation, thereby holding the light of wisdom to illuminate the darkness.

Illuminating Our Dark Corners

I once heard the statement that fear is a friend who knocks at our door to bring us another part of ourselves, a part that—on the soul level—we invited into our lives to help us become more wholly who we are. *Hmm,* I remember thinking when I understood the implications of this idea. *That is a novel way to view the situation—another piece of myself ... that I, in my greater wisdom, asked for? Yes, I can see how being whole means that all dark corners necessarily want to be brought to light ... enlightened!* I have found that when I apply this way of viewing life, it proves itself to me. I am taken out of pain and into a deeper understanding of myself. Things make sense and I better understand how my life operates on an energetic level.

A little story comes to mind—one that surprised me and illuminated some dark corners I didn't know were there. In 1997 I wrote my first book, *Fly Like a Butterfly: Yoga for Children*. The stars of the book were children aged three to nine who attended my son's Montessori school, where I had been teaching yoga for several years. Ram Das was one of those stars. He was six years old at the time, and had grown up with yoga from day one.

The photo shoot was going along smoothly. The camera was aligned with the children's sitting spot indicated by a piece of tape on the smooth, white sheets that draped the entire studio as a backdrop. Each of the children demonstrated the postures they had been practicing for months. Then the moment came for Ram Das to be photographed. He began cavorting around the stage, rumpling the sheets, doing cartwheels, and jumping and tumbling as though he had never heard the word *yoga* in his life!

My frustration quickly sparked into anger. I began commanding him. He responded with defiance, and the situation escalated from there. Losing all sense of neutrality, my "emotional mother" mind added fuel to my fury; all the other times he had been uncooperative, all the negative feedback I had ever gotten about him, came barreling down like an avalanche picking up speed and mass along the way. Then the future reared its ugly head—how was he ever going to have a happy and successful life if he refused to cooperate time and again?

As the barrage of thoughts and feelings tumbled around inside me, there was a growing awareness that I knew another way. I hit the inner pause button, and in a matter of milliseconds it dawned on me that I could call on my Self, and that letting my Self lead the way was the only way out. I listened for the sound of clarity … my Self. The internal dialogue, despite lasting just a few seconds, was something like this:

Self (kindly but firmly): *What is really going on here? Seems like anger, but what's underneath it?*

Instantly I knew the answer. Underneath the anger was fear that my one and only child would not appear in my precious first book. And with a jolt, I knew the real source of my fear: attachment—attachment to my idea of the way things should be.

Self again: *Well, you are just going to have to give that up. Because you don't know! You don't know what will happen. You cannot control this situation, but you absolutely can do something about the way you are approaching it.*

Immediately there was relief, like a deep exhalation, a surrendering into what life was presenting to me. *Okay, this may not happen* was the thought that accompanied the sensation. And once I dropped my belief in how it "should be," the stranglehold was loosened. I felt decidedly lighter, freer, and clearer.

"Ram Das," I said, my tone much more even and friendly than a moment before, "let's go into the other room for a minute and sit down at the table." We sat across from each other, his face steeling for a fight and mine still softening in the freedom of having nothing to lose, since I had let go of attachment and, with it, all expectations.

As I looked into his face, I saw not a child of mine, but a person who had his own sense of dignity. Simultaneously, I could see the child too—the child who was doing what he thought he must in order to defend himself. It was all so complicated—and so fascinating. I saw it all in this one little moment ... this moment that was so intricately woven into two people's lives, and yet it stood perfectly on its own as this one moment in time.

I still remember the words that came out of my mouth. They came from a place of trust. Trust that he absolutely knew what to do in front of the camera. Trust that he absolutely had the ability to live up to my expectations. Trust, also, that he had absolute free will. And trust that, in truth, I did not need anything from him—that it was perfect if he did and perfect if he didn't.

I looked at him with a relaxed smile in my eyes. His eyes registered the change in mine. I felt who I really knew him to be. I could almost see a beam of light shine from my heart to his as I said, "Ram Das, I know you know exactly what to do in there. So I trust that you can take care of it yourself."

He got it. He got the energetic message as well as the words. Immediately he went back to his happy-go-lucky six-year-old self, jumped down from the seat with an "Okay! See ya!" and ran into the room. I sat there, satisfied that I had gotten myself into a space of inner alignment, and recalled the feeling of the beam of light conveying the true message and bridging the distance between us. There was no sense of attachment to the outcome, no hoping the photo shoot would go "my" way. I didn't even ask the photographer how the shoot went.

A week later, the photos came back from the lab. As I came upon the photos of Ram Das, a wide smile came over my face. There he was, doing exactly what he had practiced, but with a flair that I doubt could have been achieved if I had been in the room. One of the photos was particularly spectacular. He was doing Frog Hops and the camera had caught him suspended for all time in midair, with the most joyful expression on his face.

And which photo do you think the publisher wanted for the cover? No need for a second guess!

Stepping Stones for Troubled Water

Once you come into the luminous space where you see the unseen, it is as if the unseen sees you. This means that once you allow yourself and the situation to be as it is, you project trust in the goodness of life, the unknown or the unseen. Inner clarity shines through to guide you one step at a time across troubled waters. No one can tell you what your process will be, and you may not see the next rock to guide you across rushing waters of emotion until you've stepped securely onto the first rock. Because life is fluid and malleable according to your vibrational stance, the steps can take on a variety of forms. Step by step, the radiant path lights up. Here is one way that it might look:

- **Step one:** Begin where you are, and befriend yourself as you are. You can do this by letting yourself feel the sensation that arises in response to the situation. Allow yourself to sit with the uncomfortable emotion, knowing that in doing so you allow the feeling to say its piece. This is the necessary first step to finding your peace. Whatever the method, the important thing is that you find your own way to come to peace with "what is" as the first step in transformation.

- **Step two:** Focus on small actions in "just this moment." Follow the natural impulses you may have to soothe yourself on the spot, such as yawning, rubbing the belly, touching the face or eyes, or stretching the body. Close your eyes and take a few slow, deep breaths with awareness of how they feel in your body. Drink a glass of water slowly and consciously to calm the nervous system. Deliberately put yourself in an environment where you usually feel good. Pet your cat or your dog, and appreciate the loving energy between you. If it feels good, spend time walking or running in nature, listening to the birds, the wind, taking in the colors and shapes of the natural world. Or it might feel right to go to your favorite shops and browse, or dance, or read a really good book. Whatever you choose, do it deliberately. Be focused on self-healing and reestablishing your inner spiritual alignment.

- **Step three:** In conjunction with step two, begin with positive self-talk. Find thoughts that you know are true for you that feel good when you think them. They will bring you closer into alignment with your soul or authentic Self. You might even journal your self-talk. You might write, *I know what it feels like to be centered and connected to my soul. I have done it before and I can do it again. I trust myself and I trust the flow of life to bring the best solution for me.* And perhaps followed by, *This situation has presented itself to me before, and now I feel more ready than ever to move through it. It will feel so good to release my anxiety around this. I am looking forward to it!* Positive self-talk is one of the most healing ways to uplift yourself, and you can do it at any time!

• **Step four:** As best you can, let go of the issue and trust that it is being taken care of by what you may think of as Divine Intelligence, Great Spirit, God, or what I sometimes like to call the "Universal Manager." If you are having trouble letting go, you can diffuse the energy around the issue by focusing on something that makes you feel good. You can draw comfort and encouragement from the thought that the Law of Attraction is powerfully and magnetically bringing exactly what you are vibrating.

These stepping stones over troubled water allow the issues to deactivate and make space for new, creative solutions to arise. No matter what steps you choose, being kind to yourself and connecting with what feels good for you will enhance your ability to come into your radiant, authentic Self. Then, in your radiance, you hold a space of light and healing for others. It can extend out as a prayer field for the whole world.

Raising the Lantern for the Next Generation

In the work I do with Radiant Child Yoga, I meet hundreds of inspiring and inspired Lightworkers each year. I say Lightworkers, because it is a more accurate description of the work these people are doing in the world. Yes, it is yoga. Yes, it is mindfulness, and it is meditation. But beyond any method or technique these dedicated souls are using, the real power of transformation comes from ordinary individuals holding a space of light and love for the future of our world, beginning with one child at a time. Here are a couple small glimpses of those who hold the lantern high for young people.

Karen is a high school health and physical education teacher, as well as a yoga teacher, who works with about a hundred teens each year. When each new group comes in, she always ponders, *How do I teach meaningful, transformative, healthy living skills within the somewhat limiting framework of public education models?* Karen's always in pursuit of how she can get her expansive, creative, and ever-changing ideas of natural health and mental wellness to fit in the school structure. There is no way to do this without involving the young people whom she's teaching, so at the beginning of the year, she'll ask them:

- Why are you here?
- Do you have any fears about the coming school year?
- What do you want to learn?

Through these questions, the picture becomes clearer and she becomes more insightful about how she can achieve the results she wants.

Children of all ages, including teens, are more open to adults who are in an authentic state of Self, living mindfully and practicing what they teach their students. Karen gets so much joy out of sharing the tools that have blessed her life: yoga and meditation, art, healthy eating, walking in nature, writing, and practicing present moment awareness. This beautiful combination of healthy lifestyle tools reminds Karen of many beams of light, swirling along, gently carrying the students with it and planting the seeds to help them receive a meaningful internal experience. Once those seeds are planted, Karen remembers this: we don't keep digging them up to see if they are growing! They are there and they shall grow when they are ready.

Through Karen's approach with her students, she has been able to have an impact on their lives beyond their high school years. The proof is in the responses from these young, brilliant minds. Some of her students who lean toward depression, anger, or anxiety have thanked her for the change they feel since her class. Karen trusts that the spark of light ignited in her wellness class can be a raised lantern, in some small or large way, into their future.

No good effort is wasted. It travels on the vibration of its intention and resounds in the lives it touches. As Paulo Coelho wrote in his book *The Alchemist*, "When you want something, all the universe conspires in helping you to achieve it." The question is, *do you live as if you know that small and large miracles are at work every day?*

I have a friend who has been teaching Kundalini yoga as long as I have. Her passion is to share yoga and the teachings of awareness with children who live in low-income areas. For the past fifteen years, my friend has been holding the vision of what miracles lay in the minds and hearts of these children, and how she can help to birth those miracles.

One of her stories is about a young man, a former student, who came back to see her a few years after graduating from high school. He gave her a strong hug and said, "If it wasn't for the yoga you taught me, not only would I have dropped out of school, but I am sure I would be dead or in prison by now, like so many kids I know. The way you believed in me and gave me yoga that helped me to believe in me ... well ma'am, you saved my life, of that I am sure."

***

Radiating the Frequency of Peace

As many parents and teachers have shown in their stories, children are often the catalyst for deep change within us, and as we transform ourselves, we have the opportunity to pay it forward to uplift the world.

How can I, as one human being, help our world? Can I create a vibrational frequency of peace within myself that radiates outward and affects our entire world? Is that even possible?

Our world and our minds are made of the same stuff—energy. Science is now beginning to be able to document nonphysical forces. From Gregg Braden's book *The Isaiah Effect: Decoding the Lost Science* of *Prayer and Prophecy* comes this experiment: "In a report from the third annual conference of the International Society for the Study of Subtle Energies and Energy Medicine, scientists documented the nonphysical force of emotion *actually changing* the physical molecule of DNA. ... The study reported that "individuals trained in generating focused feelings of deep love … were able to *intentionally cause a change* in the conformation [shape] of the DNA."[15]

Many people are waking up from a long sleep because events of cataclysmic proportions are taking place on our planet almost daily. It can easily feel as though we don't have power to do anything about the way our world is headed, that we can only stand by helplessly and watch the deterioration and destruction of what we love. But many, many people I meet and speak with are rising to the challenge of these times. I believe that the tide is turning, and that every day more of us are using a greater portion of our vibratory energy to be a lighthouse for peace, and what we call miracles are on the cusp of becoming everyday reality.

In response to wanting to stay connected to my wise, authentic Self through all the changes our world is going through, I created a guided practice to help me stay in balance and remember that I am—that we all are—powerful creators. When I do this practice, I feel that I am doing my part to create an energetic space of peace in our world. I hope that you and your children find that this practice blesses you and blesses the world, too.

Peace in Our Hearts, Peace in Our World: A Practice

As you read this practice, or record it and listen to it, be in a meditative space. Treat it as a meditation, or a time for prayer or contemplation. Go slowly and let the feeling and ideas sink in. To stay present, it may be helpful to be aware of your breath. If you are reading this, close your eyes after each section. Give a pause to let the words sink in.

Since children are powerful, tuned-in creators, I've included wording in more childlike language in italics after the adult sections of the practice. Feel free to improvise and adapt this for your personal use. After completing the exercise, allow a space for your child to talk about what he or she experienced. This is very subtle and sensitive work, so go slowly and focus on feeling the words resonate within you.

---

15. Gregg Braden, *The Isaiah Effect: Decoding the Lost Science of Prayer and Prophecy* (New York: Three Rivers Press, 2000), p. 219.

Sit down on the floor in a meditative position, or sit straight in a chair. If you are doing the practice with children, sit side by side or across from each other.

1. **For adults:** "I let myself relax into a state of feeling for all who are suffering, and that feeling extends out to the whole world. I allow the pain. I sit with it and let it be as it is, in trust, simply because it is part of All That Is. After some time, I find the pain has subtly transformed into something else: a compassionate healing, an accepting of the higher wisdom in this, as all, actions."

   For children: "Let's close our eyes and allow whatever we feel, even if it is sad, or angry, or fearful. If pictures come to you, things that you've seen on TV, heard people talking about, whatever it is, just let it be. It cannot hurt you to let it be. Give yourself permission to feel, and just watch what happens if you don't block your feelings."

2. **For adults:** "I feel my prayer field, my energy field, extending out in front of me and all around me. It is a beacon of light that holds a space for a bright future, a world in which all conflict is resolved in the highest manner. I don't use my rational mind to think of strategies that would resolve it. Rather, I create a space— an emptiness that contains all possibilities—in which the universal wisdom can fully work. I trust humanity. I visualize us at our best, with full awareness of the consequences of our actions, using challenges as opportunities to propel our world into a new way of being. This does not mean that those who have hurt others are not called to account, but I see this happening in the miraculous ways of the universe rather than in ways that creates more suffering and retaliation."

   For children: "Instead of trying to think about all the problems and solutions that are being talked about in our world right now, let's do something really different. Let's imagine a big, bright emptiness that stretches out in front of us, and all around us, and goes into the future. That big emptiness is a space of light in which anything is possible! Magical things, miraculous things, things no one ever thought about can all happen in this wonderful emptiness that we are allowing to be there."

3. **For adults:** "I have the courage to go into the mind and heart of someone who has hurt others. I feel the pain that can be translated into hatred and inflicting pain on others. I feel it pass through me, and I allow it as part of All That Is. I remember that when I accept what is, it cannot stay the same. My acceptance of it creates a kind of "vibrational hug" around it, and it melts. I have a sense that these beings are brought into the fold of humanity through the transformation that happens through this compassionate act."

For children: "It takes courage to go into a place inside you where you allow yourself to feel the pain that is inside a person you don't like or who has hurt you, or someone else, in some way. Think of anyone who is like that for you, and now allow them into your heart and feel their heart, too. The hate melts, and what is left is just a human being who didn't know how to handle their painful feelings."

4. **For adults:** "I trust that All That Is will unfold the events of the future that will match the vibratory frequency that I, and many others together, are holding and projecting—a sacred space where peace and truth prevail. In this deep space of trust and knowing, I feel the ecstasy that is my birthright, and I extend that birthright out to all of humanity."

For children: "Without even thinking, we trust that we will have another breath, and another, and another, right? Now let's have that same kind of trust that something good is happening, something that is connecting us with everyone else on our planet. Feel the light of peace in your heart and connect it up with everyone else, people you know and people you don't know. Let's grow peace so it stretches all around the world."

5. **Adults and children together with hands at the heart center:** "And now let's send a blessing to all the people, animals, and plants on our beautiful Mother Earth by saying together three times, "Peace to all, life to all, love to all.""

Chapter Highlights

- **We are made of light energy:** Eastern and Western science agree that at our most fundamental level, we are made of light. Chakras are the yoga term for whirling centers of light energy within our bodies as well as around us in the form of individual energy fields.

- **Children's chakras have patterns of development that change as they mature:** Being aware of this enables us to be compassionate toward them and help them stay in balance.

- **Holding the light means we trust the best in each other, and we trust universal wisdom to deliver the rest of what we are asking for:** We help children best when we approach their needs from a place of love and trust, not only in them but also in the basic goodness and wisdom of the universe.

- **Trust your process:** When you don't know how to make it all work out, just take the first step. Once you take that first step, the next one lights up.

- **Small and large miracles are happening every day:** Being a lighthouse for children is a great way to live a life filled with so much positive synchronicity that it feels miraculous.

- **Children hold the future in their young hands:** With that understanding, we as adults have the unique opportunity to shape a bright future where all living beings on Mother Earth are honored and loved.

EPILOGUE
In the Hands of the Universe

Life is a co-creative experience. When we befriend ourselves, our children learn that this is the natural way to live. When we see the level at which our children are able to live in their wisdom, we are inspired to do the same. Through learning from each other, we are born together; the parent is born through the child and the teacher is born through the student.

In our lives with children, challenges naturally occur. If we are open to it, challenges can be seen as deeper questions. Questions bring answers into focus. Answers bring a new vantage point. The new vantage point leads to new challenges and new questions, and so the beautiful cycle of growing into our Self continues.

To understand the phenomenon of co-creation is to realize that we are co-creating with the entire universe. You might say that in the hands of the universe, the unseen becomes seen. What we term a "miracle" begins to become normal life.

A family begins meditating together every evening, and it becomes the catalyst for tremendous positive change in their daily lives. A teacher sees the potential in her student, and he begins to go beyond anyone's expectations. A mother surrenders to her child becoming a young man, and he shares his grown-up wisdom with her. All these miracles, large and small, are born from powerful and prayerful intentions. They are visions that come to life in the hands of the universe, All That Is, and so the co-creation continues.

Most importantly, let's share our high heart and our authenticity every day with the children in our care. Let's see their innate wisdom guiding them along through every challenge and every joy. Can you imagine a world filled with children who grow up knowing who they are? Can you imagine their children, and the generations that follow? What a phenomenal reality we are creating from our vision!

I thank you for allowing me this time and space to share with you. I leave these pages with a poem I wrote, from my heart to yours.

Ending/Beginning

The next curve in the path,

the next juncture,

the next point of growth,

is coming, I know,

because it is never-ending.

Whatever it is,

I accept it with joy

as I remember

that it brings me more of myself

to be,

to share,

to serve the world

in Love.

To All That Is,

the God of All,

in All as All,

this soul gratefully bows.

Resources

Books, DVDs, CDs, and Cards by Shakta Khalsa

Fly Like a Butterfly: Yoga for Children, Sterling Publishing
(rights have reverted to author)

K.I.S.S. Guide to Yoga, DK Publishing

Kundalini Yoga, DK Publishing

Yoga for Women, DK Publishing

Yoga in Motion DVD

Cozy CD

Happy CD

Present Moment Awareness CD

Yoga Warrior Cards

Other Relevant Resources

Ask and It Is Given, Esther and Jerry Hicks, Hay House

The Brain That Changes Itself, Norman Doidge, MD, Penguin Books

Hands of Light, Barbara Ann Brennan, Bantam Books

How to Talk So Kids Will Listen & Listen So Kids Will Talk, Adele Faber
and Elaine Mazlish, Avon Books

The Isaiah Effect: Decoding the Lost Science of Prayer and Prophecy, Gregg
Braden, Three Rivers Press

Loving What Is, Byron Katie, Random House
Playing in the Unified Field, Carla Hannaford, PhD, Great River Books
The Power of Now, Eckhart Tolle, New World Library

To Write to the Author

If you wish to contact the author or would like more information about this book, please write to the author in care of Llewellyn Worldwide Ltd. and we will forward your request. Both the author and the publisher appreciate hearing from you and learning of your enjoyment of this book and how it has helped you. Llewellyn Worldwide Ltd. cannot guarantee that every letter written to the author can be answered, but all will be forwarded. Please write to:

Shakta Khalsa
℅ Llewellyn Worldwide
2143 Wooddale Drive
Woodbury, MN 55125-2989

Please enclose a self-addressed stamped envelope for reply,
or $1.00 to cover costs. If outside the U.S.A., enclose
an international postal reply coupon.

Many of Llewellyn's authors have websites with additional information and resources. For more information, please visit our website at http://www.llewellyn.com

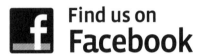
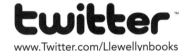

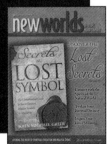